Psychodynamic Approaches to Psychopathology, Vol 1

Editors

RACHEL Z. RITVO
SCHUYLER W. HENDERSON

CHILD AND ADOLESCENT PSYCHIATRIC CLINICS OF NORTH AMERICA

www.childpsych.theclinics.com

Consulting Editor
HARSH K. TRIVEDI

January 2013 • Volume 22 • Number 1

ELSEVIER

Elsevier Inc. • 1600 John F. Kennedy Boulevard • Suite 1800 • Philadelphia, Pennsylvania 19103-2899

http://www.childpsych.theclinics.com

CHILD AND ADOLESCENT PSYCHIATRIC CLINICS OF NORTH AMERICA Volume 22, Number 1
January 2013 ISSN 1056–4993, ISBN-13: 978-1-4557-7071-7

Editor: Joanne Husovski
Developmental Editor: Donald Mumford

Child and Adolescent Psychiatric Clinics of North America (ISSN 1056-4993) is published quarterly by Elsevier Inc., 360 Park Avenue South, New York, NY 10010-1710. Months of issue are January, April, July, and October. Business and Editorial Offices: 1600 John F. Kennedy Boulevard, Suite 1800, Philadelphia, PA 19103-2899. Periodicals postage paid at New York, NY and additional mailing offices. Subscription prices are $297.00 per year (US individuals), $453.00 per year (US institutions), $150.00 per year (US students), $343.00 per year (Canadian individuals), $546.00 per year (Canadian institutions), $190.00 per year (Canadian students), $408.00 per year (international individuals), $546.00 per year (international institutions), and $190.00 per year (international students). International air speed delivery is included in all *Clinics* subscription prices. All prices are subject to change without notice. **POSTMASTER:** Send address changes to *Child and Adolescent Psychiatric Clinics of North America*, Elsevier Health Sciences Division, Subscription Customer Service, 3251 Riverport Lane, Maryland Heights, MO 63043. **Customer Service: 1-800-654-2452 (U.S. and Canada); 314-447-8871 (outside U.S. and Canada). Fax: 314-447-8029. E-mail: JournalsCustomerService-usa@elsevier.com (for print support) or journalsonlinesupport-usa@elsevier.com (for online support).**

Reprints. For copies of 100 or more of articles in this publication, please contact the Commercial Reprints Department, Elsevier Inc., 360 Park Avenue South, New York, New York 10010-1710 Tel.: (212) 633-3812; Fax: (212) 462-1935, e-mail: reprints@elsevier.com.

Child and Adolescent Psychiatric Clinics of North America is covered in *MEDLINE/PubMed (Index Medicus), ISI, SSCI, Research Alert, Social Search, Current Contents,* and *EMBASE/Excerpta Medica.*

Printed and bound by CPI Group (UK) Ltd, Croydon, CR0 4YY

Transferred to digital print 2012

Contributors

CONSULTING EDITOR

HARSH K. TRIVEDI, MD
Associate Professor of Psychiatry, Vanderbilt University School of Medicine; Executive Medical Director, and Chief of Staff, Vanderbilt Psychiatric Hospital, Nashville, Tennessee

CONSULTING EDITOR EMERITUS

ANDRÉS MARTIN, MD, MPH

FOUNDING CONSULTING EDITOR

MELVIN LEWIS, MBBS, FRCPSYCH, DCH

GUEST EDITORS

RACHEL Z. RITVO, MD
Assistant Clinical Professor of Psychiatry and Behavioral Sciences, George Washington University School of Medicine and Health Sciences, Washington, DC

SCHUYLER W. HENDERSON, MD, MPH
Assistant Clinical Professor of Psychiatry, Department of Child and Adolescent Psychiatry, New York University, New York, New York

AUTHORS

SIMON CREGEEN, BA Hons, MPsychPsych
Consultant Child and Adolescent Psychotherapist, Central Manchester University Hospitals NHS Foundation Trust, United Kingdom; Programme Director, MSc in Developmental Psychology and Clinical Practice, Anna Freud Centre, London, United Kingdom

IDA DANCYGER, PhD
Clinical Associate Professor of Psychology in Psychiatry, Hofstra North Shore-LIJ School of Medicine, Hempstead, New York; Psychologist, Division of Child and Adolescent Psychiatry, Department of Psychiatry, Zucker Hillside Hospital, Glen Oaks, New York

VICTOR FORNARI, MD
Professor of Psychiatry, Hofstra North Shore-LIJ School of Medicine, Hempstead, New York; Director, Division of Child and Adolescent Psychiatry, Department of Psychiatry, Zucker Hillside Hospital, Glen Oaks, New York

ANDREW J. GERBER, MD, PhD
Assistant Professor of Clinical Psychiatry, Division of Child and Adolescent Psychiatry, New York State Psychiatric Institute, Columbia University, New York, New York

CAROL HUGHES, BA (Psych)
Consultant Child and Adolescent Psychotherapist, Cambridgeshire and Peterborough NHS Trust, United Kingdom; Anna Freud Centre, London, United Kingdom

SCOTT KRAKOWER, DO
Fellow, Child and Adolescent Psychiatry, Hofstra North Shore-LIJ School of Medicine, Hempstead, New York; Division of Child and Adolescent Psychiatry, Zucker Hillside Hospital, Glen Oaks, New York

NORKA T. MALBERG, PsyD
Private Practice and Clinical Faculty, Yale Child Study Center, New Haven, Connecticut

LINDA C. MAYES, MD
Arnold Gesell Professor in the Child Study Center and Professor of Epidemiology (Chronic Diseases), of Pediatrics and of Psychology; Chair, Directorial Team, Anna Freud Centre at London; Special Advisor, Dean, Yale Child Study Center, New Haven, Connecticut

NICK MIDGLEY, BA Hons, MSc, PsychD
Child and Adolescent Psychotherapist and Programme Director, MSc in Developmental Psychology and Clinical Practice, Anna Freud Centre/University College London, London, United Kingdom

BARBARA MILROD, MD
Professor of Psychiatry, NYP Weill Cornell Medical College, New York, New York

XENIA PROTOPOPESCU, MD
Clinical Instructor, Department of Psychiatry, New York University, New York, New York

SANDRA RUSCONI-SERPA, PhD
Director of Research in Child and Adolescent Psychiatry, University of Geneva Hospitals and Faculty of Medicine; Senior Lecturer in Clinical Psychology, University of Geneva Faculty of Psychology, Social Sciences and Education, Geneva, Switzerland

MARGARET RUSTIN, BA Hons
Consultant Child and Adolescent Psychotherapist, Tavistock and Portman NHS Trust; Programme Director, MSc in Developmental Psychology and Clinical Practice, Anna Freud Centre, London, United Kingdom

DANIEL S. SCHECHTER, MD
Medical Director, Pediatric Consult-Liaison Unit and Parent-Child Research, Child and Adolescent Psychiatry Service (SPEA); Senior Lecturer in Psychiatry, University of Geneva Hospitals and Faculty of Medicine, Geneva, Switzerland

ARIANE SCHWAB, MD
Chief Resident and Post-graduate Fellow, Pediatric Consult-Liaison Unit, Child and Adolescent Psychiatry Service (SPEA), University of Geneva Hospitals and Faculty of Medicine, Geneva, Switzerland

THEODORE SHAPIRO, MD
NYP Weill Cornell Medical College, New York, New York

GABRIELLE SILVER, MD
Assistant Professor of Psychiatry, Director of Child and Adolescent Psychiatry Consultation Services to Pediatrics, Department of Psychiatry, NYP Weill Cornell Medical College, New York, New York

LENORE C. TERR, MD
Clinical Professor of Psychiatry, Department of Psychiatry, Langley Porter Institute, University of California San Francisco School of Medicine, San Francisco, California

Contents

CHILD AND ADOLESCENT PSYCHIATRIC CLINICS

FORTHCOMING ISSUES

Psychodynamic Treatment Approaches to Psychopathology, vol 2
Rachel Z. Ritvo, MD, and
Schuyler W. Henderson, MD,
Guest Editors

Complementary and Integrative Therapies
Deborah Simkin, MD, and
Charles Popper, MD,
Guest Editors

Psychosis
Jean Frazier, MD, and
Yael Dvir, MD, *Guest Editors*

RECENT ISSUES

October 2012
Psychopharmacology
Harsh K. Trivedi, MD, and
Kiki D. Chang, MD, *Guest Editors*

July 2012
Anxiety Disorders
Moira Rynn, MD, Hilary Vidair, PhD, and
Jennifer Urbano Blackford, PhD,
Guest Editors

April 2012
Child and Adolescent Depression
Stuart J. Goldman, MD, and
Frances Wren, MD, *Guest Editors*

January 2012
Evidence-Based School Psychiatry
Jeffrey Q. Bostic, MD, EdD, and
Alexa L. Bagnell, MD, FRCPC,
Guest Editors

A Fresh Look at Psychodynamic Approaches to Psychopathology in Children and Adolescents

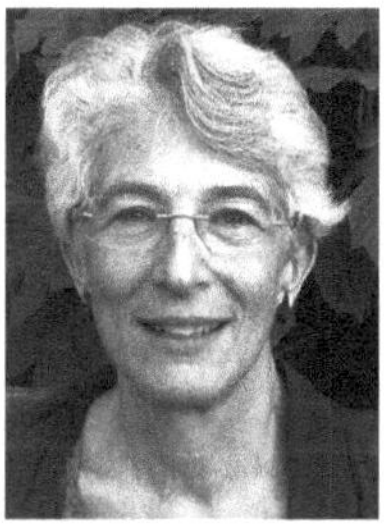

Rachel Z. Ritvo, MD *and* Schuyler W. Henderson, MD, MPH
Guest Editors

This issue of *Child and Adolescent Psychiatric Clinics of North America* is the first of two devoted to updating our colleagues on developments in psychodynamic psychotherapy for children and adolescents. A century has passed since child psychotherapy made its debut with Sigmund Freud's 1909 publication of "Analysis of a Phobia in a Five-Year-Old Boy,"[1] known to most child and adolescent psychiatrists as the case of "Little Hans." *Child and Adolescent Psychiatric Clinics of North America* last took a close look at psychodynamic psychotherapy in 1997.[2] Now, in 2013, although the compilation of articles in 2 volumes of *Child and Adolescent Psychiatric Clinics of North America* has not exhausted the breadth of research and scholarship in contemporary child and adolescent psychodynamic psychiatry, they have brought together emerging empirical research in psychodynamic psychotherapy while culling the classical literature for the tried and true of the clinical psychodynamic knowledge base.

This issue, "Psychodynamic Approaches to Psychopathology," focuses on the psychodynamic understanding of the child and adolescent in both the broad terms of neurobiology and development and, more narrowly, the dynamic forces underpinning specific clinical conditions. While 20th century psychodynamic psychiatry was grounded primarily on clinical case studies and the passage of the psychotherapeutic craft from teacher to student, this volume highlights the efforts of researchers to bring empirical tools to the study and treatment of psychopathology in children and adolescents. For this issue and the one that follows, neither the editors nor our authors have limited themselves to the work of Americans. Much of the new and exciting research on psychodynamics is taking place across The Pond, in the United Kingdom and Europe.

Protopopescu and Gerber kick off the current volume with their article, "Bridging the Gap Between Neuroscientific and Psychodynamic Models of Mind." Limited by the tools of 19th century neurology, Freud abandoned his "Project for a Scientific Psychology" in 1896,[3] giving up his attempt to explain the mind in terms of neuronal processes. Throughout the 20th century psychoanalysis let the effort lie fallow, but

Child Adolesc Psychiatric Clin N Am 22 (2013) ix–xii
http://dx.doi.org/10.1016/j.chc.2012.09.001 childpsych.theclinics.com

now, in the 21st century, advances in neuroimaging, molecular biology, and genetics allow considerable insight into the biological mechanisms that account for mental activity. Protopopescu and Gerber tackle the difficult task of reconciling the neuroscientific and psychodynamic models of mind. Deeply versed in both fields, they are able to point out fertile bridging concepts, schemas, for example, as well as the pitfalls inherent in too simplistic a view of either field. They have collected for *Child and Adolescent Psychiatric Clinics of North America* readers, in 2 comprehensive tables accompanying the article, the neuroimaging studies of psychotherapy effects on brain function and a summary of key brain regions for mental functions.

"The Contemporary Psychodynamic Developmental Perspective," presented by Malberg and Mayes, retains, but also moves beyond, the classical concepts of libidinal stages and developmental lines. They emphasize the role of empirically based attachment theory in the transformation of the psychodynamic developmental perspective from a 1-person perspective to a dyadic, intersubjective perspective. Their approach to developmental theory is integrative: integrating earlier psychoanalytic theories with newer theories; integrating theory and research from multiple disciplines; and integrating a focus on the individual with a systemic view of the individual functioning within a social environment.

For today's child and adolescent psychiatrist, much of the clinical wisdom of 20th century child and adolescent psychoanalysis is difficult to access for 3 reasons:

- First, the language of psychiatry has shifted and much of the psychoanalytic terminology is unfamiliar and confusing to readers today.
- Second, the focus of child and adolescent mental health practice of the first three-quarters of the 20th century was largely on adjustment and maladjustment of patients rather than on treating specific diagnoses. Although psychodynamic practitioners developed formulations for prominent symptom groups such as depression and anxiety, they rarely gathered this information under these labels. Typical psychodynamic formulations are passed on in supervision but can be difficult to locate in the literature. With the advent of DSM III in the 1980s, while psychodynamic clinicians clung to the adjustment disorders for diagnostic labeling, the mainstream of child and adolescent psychiatry and psychology moved toward matching treatments to the array of Axis I diagnostic categories. In this issue the selection of articles to address specific conditions includes both the diagnosis-specific approach and the adaptational view.
- Third, psychodynamic psychotherapy has lagged in embracing the quantitative empirical research methods that allow therapeutic interventions to compete in the evidence-based medicine culture of the past 2 decades. Fortunately, psychodynamic researchers have emerged in recent years who are taking up this challenge, although the costs of such a research agenda are daunting and funding is scant to nil. In this issue we present the work of both researchers working with manualized treatments and researchers working through extensive sustained clinical observation.

Anxiety disorders and depression are very common in youth and have long been the focus of psychodynamic treatment. The Cornell team who developed manualized Panic Focused Psychodynamic Psychotherapy[4,5] bring us Silver and colleagues' article on Child and adolescent Anxiety Psychodynamic Psychotherapy (CAPP), a manualized 20- to 24-session psychodynamic psychotherapy built on the basic psychoanalytic assumption that anxiety symptoms carry specific psychological meaning reflective of underlying psychological conflicts. Midgley and coworkers offer a contemporary psychodynamic understanding of depression in adolescence as well as an overview of manualized Short-Term Psychoanalytic Psychotherapy (STPP) for adolescents 11 to 17 years old with moderate to severe depression. STPP was developed for a clinical trial currently underway in the UK—the Improving Mood with Psychoanalytic and Cognitive-Behavioral Therapy Study (IMPACT).

Bringing evidence-based medicine approaches to the treatment of eating disorders has proved challenging. In clinical practice, psychodynamic approaches remain an important component of the treatment for young people with eating disorders. Dancyger and colleagues have written a comprehensive review of treatment studies that include psychodynamically informed therapy. Their findings suggest that further research into psychodynamically informed treatments is warranted.

Psychological recovery from trauma has long been a focus of psychodynamic thought and therapy. Beginning with her work with the children of the Chowchilla bus hijacking[6] in the 1970s, Terr has been a leader in the clinical study of the developmental variations in response to trauma and from her work has distilled 3 dynamic principles of healing that can be "fluidly mixed" with a wide range of therapeutic modalities. Schwab and coworkers turn the adaptational lens on dyads of the chronically ill children and their traumatically stressed parents. In keeping with several authors in this issue of *Child and Adolescent Psychiatric Clinics of North America,* they introduce the reader to the power of the concept of mentalization, its observable expression in reflective function, and its use in clinical interventions.

This issue and its companion issue owe a debt to the Norbert and Charlotte Rieger Foundation, which, for the past decade, has supported a psychodynamic psychotherapy paper prize at the American Academy of Child and Adolescent Psychiatry. Several authors in these volumes have been recipients of this award. Working on promotion for the award brought the editors of these volumes together and made clear to us that there were ample developments in psychodynamic psychotherapy for children and adolescents to support the production of this issue of the *Child and Adolescent Psychiatric Clinics of North America* and its companion.

Mentalization, play, parent work, family therapy, the psychodynamic approach to psychopharmacology, and a thorough review of psychodynamic psychotherapy outcome studies are the topics for the subsequent issue of *Child and Adolescent Psychiatric Clinics of North America*, "Psychodynamic Psychotherapy Treatment Modalities for Children and Adolescents."

Rachel Z. Ritvo, MD
George Washington University School of Medicine and Health Sciences
Washington, DC, USA

Schuyler W. Henderson, MD, MPH
Department of Child and Adolescent Psychiatry
New York University
New York, New York, USA

E-mail addresses:
rzritvomd@gmail.com (R.Z. Ritvo)
schuylermd@yahoo.com (S.W. Henderson)

REFERENCES

1. Freud S. Analysis of a phobia in a five-year-old boy (1909). In: Strachey JE, editor. The standard edition of the complete psychological works of Sigmund Freud, vol. X. London: Hogarth Press; 1955. p. 3–149.

2. Freud S. Project for a scientific psychology (1950 [1895]). In: Strachey J, editor. Pre-psycho-analytic publications and unpublished drafts (1886-1899), vol. I. London: Hogarth Press; 1966. p. 281–397.
3. Milrod B, Busch F, Cooper AM, et al. Manual of panic-focused psychodynamic psychotherapy. Washington, DC: American Psychiatric Press, Inc; 1997.
4. Milrod B, Busch F, Shapiro T. Psychodynamic approaches to the adolescent with panic disorder. Malabar (FL): Krieger Publishing Company; 2004.
5. O'Brien JD. Psychotherapy. Child Adolesc Psychiatr Clin N Am 1997;6(1).
6. Terr LC. Children of Chowchilla. Psychoanal Study Child 1979;34:552–632.

Bridging the Gap Between Neuroscientific and Psychodynamic Models in Child and Adolescent Psychiatry

Xenia Protopopescu, MD[a], Andrew J. Gerber, MD, PhD[b,*]

KEYWORDS

- Neuroscience • Neuroimaging • Psychodynamic • Psychiatry • Child
- Development

KEY POINTS

- Neuroimaging demonstrates measurable changes in brain function after psychotherapy, and interpretation of these often-complex results requires a productive dialogue among neuroscientists and psychodynamic clinicians and theorists.
- Neuroimaging, molecular biology, and genetics have significant contributions to make in elucidating the biologic mechanisms that account for mental activity.
- Schemas are a crucial bridging concept for neuroscience and psychodynamic models of the mind, and are described by a growing body of empiric literature.

INTRODUCTION

Critics of those who synthesize psychodynamic theory and neuroscience have pointed out that relying on a biologic perspective limits the significance of psychodynamic contributions, and that psychodynamic insights can be distorted by trying to fit them within a scientific framework.[1,2] Psychodynamic theorists have expressed concern that the richness and complexity of psychodynamic theory will be lost in experimental assessments.[3] At the same time, psychodynamic clinicians and theorists have been accused of neglecting insights from neuroscience and failing to engage in systematic hypothesis testing.[4,5]

Funding Sources: Dr Gerber: New York State Psychiatric Institute, Columbia University, Sackler Institute for Psychobiology. Dr Protopopescu: NewYork-Presbyterian Hospital.
Conflicts of Interest: Dr Gerber: Grant support from Eli Lilly via the American Academy of Child and Adolescent Psychiatry and Forest Research Laboratories. Dr Protopopescu: Nothing to Disclose.
[a] Department of Psychiatry, New York University, 1 Park Avenue, 8th floor, New York, NY 10016, USA; [b] Division of Child and Adolescent Psychiatry, New York State Psychiatric Institute, Columbia University, 1051 Riverside Drive, Unit 74, New York, NY 10032, USA
* Corresponding author. Department of Psychiatry, New York State Psychiatric Institute, 1051 Riverside Drive, Unit 74, New York, NY 10032.
E-mail address: gerbera@nyspi.columbia.edu

Child Adolesc Psychiatric Clin N Am 22 (2013) 1–31
http://dx.doi.org/10.1016/j.chc.2012.08.008 **childpsych.theclinics.com**
1056-4993/13/$ – see front matter

Abbreviations: Neuroscience and Psychodynamic Models in Child and Adolescent Psychiatry	
ABL	Amygdale basolateral nucleus
ACC	Anterior cingulate cortex
ASD	Autism spectrum disorders
BDNF	Brain-derived neurotrophic growth factor
CA	Central nucleus amygdala
DA	Dopaminergic
DLPFC	Dorsolateral prefrontal cortex
dmPFC	Dorsomedial prefrontal cortex
FFA	Fusiform face area
HPA	Hypothalamic-pituitary-adrenal
MDD	Major depressive disorder
mOFC	Medial orbitofrontal cortex
mPFC	Medial prefrontal cortex
OFC	Orbitofrontal cortex
PFC	Prefrontal cortex
pMFC	Posterior medial frontal cortex
PMDD	Premenstrual dysphoric disorder
RT-PQRS	Randomized controlled trial psychotherapy quality rating scale
SMA	Supplementary motor area
vmPFC	Ventromedial prefrontal cortex

Cognitive and Developmental Neuroscience

Cognitive neuroscience, fueled by neuroimaging, genetics, and molecular biology, has made tremendous strides toward elucidating the biologic mechanisms of mental activity.[6] Developmental neuroscience (exploring the processes that generate, shape, and reshape the nervous systems throughout life) is of particular interest to psychodynamic thinking, because the developmental approach to psychopathology is the traditional framework of psychoanalysis.[7,8] Psychodynamic clinicians aim to uncover the developmental stages and sequelae of psychopathology, and discover potentially therapeutic ways to influence these developmental patterns.[9] Discussions between psychodynamic child clinicians and neuroscientists have the potential to yield new insights into developmental psychopathology. Several papers have attempted to reconcile biologic and psychodynamic psychiatry,[10–13] but despite the significant need for neuroscience to be informed by comprehensive theories of mind and for psychodynamic theory to incorporate new developments in understanding the brain, several challenges exist in engaging scientists and analysts in combined efforts.

Neuroscience Techniques and Studies

Neuroscience techniques for studying the brain are constantly evolving and cover a tremendous range spatially (molecules [DNA, RNA, protein, neurotransmitters], cells [electrophysiological recordings, microscopy], neural networks [functional MRI (fMRI), positron emission tomography (PET), single-photon emission CT (SPECT), electroencephalogram, magnetoencephalogram], ecosystems [social neuroscience, epidemiology]) and temporally (millisecond molecular and electrophysiologic processes, development across the lifespan, evolution over generations). Neuroimaging (fMRI, PET, SPECT) procedures are based on the metabolic activity accompanying neural activity, which causes mental activity to generate measurable changes in blood flow, use of oxygen, and use of glucose. Statistical methods in neuroimaging are complex, and interpreting tantalizing images of neural activity without understanding methodological limitations is problematic. In one comic demonstration of this, findings were obtained from an fMRI "experiment" using the brain of a dead salmon in a social perspective–taking task when no correction for multiple comparisons was performed.[14]

In addition to complicated statistics, neuroimaging studies rely heavily on the cognitive psychology literature for the development of tasks to probe mental activity. Neuroimaging studies also make use of a vast array of comparisons (between task conditions, groups of individuals, different time points). It is common for the main finding in a neuroimaging study to involve multiple subtractions to examine conditions of interest. For example, in a study of premenstrual dysphoric disorder (PMDD), amygdala activity was noted to be increased to negative versus neutral words in subjects with PMDD versus normal controls in the premenstrual versus postmenstrual phase of the cycle.[15] It would be easy to conclude from reading the abstract of this paper that the amygdala has an exaggerated response to negative stimuli in women with PMDD when they are premenstrual. However, more nuanced reading of the results indicates that this contrast is driven by an enhanced postmenstrual amygdala response to negative words in the supernormal (woman with no premenstrual syndrome) controls as much as it is driven by increased premenstrual amygdala activity to negative words in PMDD. Such 3-tiered contrasts are typical in neuroimaging studies of psychotherapy, in which a task condition is examined in contrast to a control condition, patients are contrasted with controls, and pretreatment scans are contrasted with posttreatment scans. Any clinicians and theorists with a preliminary understanding of these techniques run the risk of overgeneral conclusions when interpreting research studies.

Individual Variability

Individual variability is a significant problem for neuroscience research. Genetically identical cells and animals have significant variability in many cellular parameters, and variable solutions producing similar phenotypes are an important substrate for evolutionary selection.[16,17] At the DNA level, nonspecificity and malleability of gene action results in considerable flexibility in the capacity of the genome to respond to diverse conditions.[16] Neuronal circuits can vary across individuals and are not optimally designed. A large body of work suggests that many "good enough" solutions that are consistent with the normal behavior of healthy animals in their usual environments.[18] The scientific process often relies on averaged results across populations (of molecules, cells, or individuals), with reconfirmation of findings noted to be essential to accumulate sufficient evidence to prove or disprove a scientific hypothesis. This dependence on consistent repetition becomes increasingly problematic as systems of increasing complexity, individual variability, and rarity are explored. The human mind is of sufficient complexity that internal variability must be considered in addition to variability between individuals.

Neuroscientists would benefit from understanding the subtleties of psychodynamic models, because imaging studies have attempted to tackle complex topics such as romantic love, maternal love, and hate through summed images of groups of subjects. Psychodynamic clinicians and theorists are experts on the tremendous individual variability in these complicated human experiences, and a detailed understanding of this variability is essential to designing intelligent paradigms for probing these phenomena in groups of subjects.

Although Tolstoy famously wrote, "All happy families resemble one another, each unhappy family is unhappy in its own way," even happiness, that supposedly simplest of human emotions, is far more complex from the perspective of a psychoanalyst. Salman Akhtar[19] has categorized happiness into 4 varieties: pleasure-based (elation), assertion-based (joy), merger-based (ecstasy), and fulfillment-based (contentment). In this model, neuroimaging the state of "happiness" may be assisted by individual assessments separating subjects experiencing different types of happiness. In addition to the important role of psychodynamic theorists in discussing intersubject variability in cognitive and emotional states, transference is another phenomenon related to scientific inquiry to which analysts can contribute a fuller understanding. Objectivity in the pursuit of understanding the human mind is difficult to achieve, and neuroscientists constantly project and anthropomorphize when attempting to understand the mechanisms of their own brains.

Freud[20] wrote:

> *So it comes about that psycho-analysis derives nothing but disadvantages from its middle position between medicine and philosophy. Doctors regard it as a speculative system and refuse to believe that, like every other natural science, it is based on a patient and tireless elaboration of facts from the world of perception; philosophers, measuring it by the standard of their own artificially constructed systems, find that it starts from impossible premises and reproach it because its most general concepts (which are only now in process of evolution) lack clarity and precision. This state of affairs is enough to account for the reluctant and hesitant reception of analysis in scientific quarters. But it does not explain the outbursts of indignation, derision, and scorn which, in disregard of every standard of logic and good taste, have characterized the controversial methods of its opponents. A reaction of such kind suggests that resistances other than purely intellectual ones were stirred up and that powerful emotional forces were aroused. And, there are indeed plenty of things to be found in the theory of psycho-analysis calculated to produce such an effect as this upon the passions of men of every kind and not of scientists alone.*

This article provides a selective review of the neuroscience and child-psychoanalytic literature, with a focus on areas of significant overlap and an emphasis on comprehensive theories in developmental neuroscience and child psychoanalysis with testable mechanisms of action. Topics include molecular biology and genetics findings relevant to psychotherapy research, neuroimaging findings relevant to psychotherapy, brain regions of interest for psychotherapy, neurobiological changes caused by psychotherapy, use of neuroimaging to predict treatment outcome, and schemas as a bridging concept between psychodynamic and cognitive neuroscience models.

MOLECULAR BIOLOGY AND GENETICS FINDINGS RELEVANT TO PSYCHOTHERAPY RESEARCH

Molecular biology and genetics have significant contributions to make in understanding the biologic mechanisms that account for mental activity.[4] Epigenetic studies providing genetic mechanisms for the transgenerational transmission of trauma are of particular interest to child psychodynamic clinicians.[21]

Overwhelming evidence from the past several decades, particularly from studies of identical versus fraternal twins, has shown that psychiatric illnesses, including depression, anxiety, bipolar disorder, schizophrenia, and autism, have a large heritable component that explains anywhere from a quarter to more than half of the variability in risk from one individual to another (depending on how these disorders are defined). Although some of this variability is accounted for by rare mutations that explain one in thousands or even millions of cases, most attention in psychiatric genetics has been devoted to so-called common variants; that is, genes that show common variability in the population and contribute, either alone or in combination, to increased or decreased risk of various psychiatric illnesses. Through studying the biologic mechanisms of these common variants at the cellular level, and then linking them to larger brain circuits as measured with neuroimaging, investigators have begun to understand the causal relationships between genetic differences and psychiatric illness.

Brain-Derived Neurotrophic Growth Factor

Brain-derived neurotrophic growth factor (BDNF) plays a critical role in nervous system development and function, and a common single nucleotide variant (or polymorphism), BDNF Val66Met, has been shown to lead to memory impairment and susceptibility to neuropsychiatric disorders in humans heterozygous for this variant. BDNF Met/Met mice showed increased anxiety-related behaviors that were not normalized with fluoxetine[22]; impairment in extinction learning that was rescued by d-cycloserine (a cognitive enhancer)[23]; and impairment in *N*-methyl-D-aspartate receptor–dependent synaptic plasticity in the hippocampus.[24] Researchers have proposed that the BDNF Val66Met mutation may impair the efficacy of selective serotonin reuptake inhibitor drug treatment through impairing fluoxetine-induced enhancement of adult hippocampus plasticity,[25] and may mediate genetic differences in ovarian steroid-related behavioral changes and disorders because it dramatically alters the fluctuation of spatial memory, hippocampal Akt phosphorylation, and PSD-95 protein expression across the estrous cycle.[26] BDNF Val66Met alters extinction learning in both mouse and human, leads to atypical frontoamygdala activity in the human brain, and may, through impairing learning of cues that signal safety versus threat, play a role in the mechanisms of anxiety disorders.[27] Efficacy of treatments, such as exposure therapy, relying on extinction mechanisms, is also likely be affected by BDNF polymorphism.

Multiple Genes for Psychopathological Phenotype

Genetic influences on psychopathology are multifactorial, with each gene generally contributing a small fraction of the risk. Gene effects that may be too subtle to capture when exploring diagnosis through gene interactions alone are often examined through intermediate phenotypes, such as amygdala reactivity, coupling of amygdala and anterior cingulate cortex activity, anterior cingulate cortex volume, hippocampal volume, and serotonin receptor 1A binding potential.[28] For example, serotonergic genes (SLC6A4, HTR1A, MAOA, TPH2) and BDNF have all been shown to influence these intermediate phenotypes.[28]

Single Gene for Multiple Psychopathologic Phenotypes

In addition to multiple genes being required for a psychopathological phenotype, one gene may influence multiple psychopathologic phenotypes. For example, the catechol-O-methyltransferase (COMT) Val158Met polymorphism, which influences neurocognitive function in schizophrenia (particularly effecting measures of processing speed and attention),[29] has also been associated with fibromyalgia,[30] increased sensitivity to pain,[31] differences in normal cognitive aging and personality traits in old age,[32] modulation of the relationship between serious life events and impulsive aggression in individuals with borderline personality disorder,[33] and contribution to negativity bias.[34] COMT Val158Met and the serotonin transporter promotor region (5HTTLPR) functional loci have been shown to interact to predict persistence of anxiety across adolescence, with carriers homozygous for both the COMT Met158 and the 5HTTLPR short alleles (Met158Met + short-short) having a more than 2-fold reduction in odds of reporting persistent generalized anxiety.[35] Schizophrenia-risk genes dysbindin 1[36] and neuregulin 1[37] have been associated with impaired verbal fluency and changes in brain activation in healthy individuals.

Genes Predict Treatment Response

Genetics can also predict treatment response; for example, COMT Met allele load predicted improvement in working memory performance and prefrontal physiology after 8 weeks of treatment with olanzapine.[38] Another gene (COMT) by drug (antipsychotic) interaction study in schizophrenia showed that the verbal IQ performance of a val/val individual was significantly lower with increasing antipsychotic medication dose, whereas this association was reversed in Met carriers.[39]

In major depressive disorder, hippocampal volumes have been associated with 5-HTTLPR and BDNF (Val66Met) polymorphisms, and increased amygdala activation has been associated with 5-HTTLPR and 5-HT1a receptor polymorphisms.[40] A neuroimaging study of dopamine D2 receptor gene polymorphism DRD2-TAQ-IA showed that A1-allele carriers with reduced dopamine D2 receptor densities learned to avoid actions with negative consequences less efficiently, and their posterior medial frontal cortex, which is involved in feedback monitoring, responded less to negative feedback.[41]

Epigenetics

Epigenetics is the study of heritable changes in gene expression or cellular phenotype caused by mechanisms other than changes in underlying DNA nucleotide sequence. DNA methylation, histone modification, chromatin modifications, and RNA methylation are examples of changes that regulate gene expression without altering the underlying DNA sequence. Increasing evidence shows epigenetic inheritance in rodents and humans, providing a mechanism whereby adverse environmental factors (toxicants, diet, postnatal care, and trauma) can affect not only the individual directly exposed to these factors but also their offspring, potentially across multiple generations.[21] Although epigenetic mechanisms seem highly likely to play an important role in the development of psychiatric illness in humans, the exact causal relationship between epigenetic mechanisms and later psychiatric diagnoses have yet to be demonstrated.

The genes mentioned here are a small subset of the growing number of genetic polymorphisms being shown to influence psychopathologic risk, cognitive function, and brain activity.

NEUROIMAGING FINDINGS RELEVANT TO PSYCHOTHERAPY

The findings of functional neuroimaging are based on having human participants complete carefully constructed tasks, usually referred to as "functional imaging paradigms" during an MRI scan designed to measure oxygenation in different parts of the brain, thus providing an indication of which sets of neurons are most active or inactive (compared with other conditions or subjects) during a particular task. A large number of these neuroimaging paradigms are relevant to psychotherapy research, such as those presenting classical conditioning, instructed fear, human faces,[42] guided imagery, scripts, and emotionally arousing stimuli (the International Affective Picture System, human speech, environmental sounds, or linguistic stimuli).

Interpreting Results From Functional Neuroimaging

Interpreting the results from neuroimaging paradigms is rarely straightforward, and requires constantly challenging assumptions about the mechanisms of the mind. Is the mind composed of highly specialized components for specific aspects of cognition, or more general-purpose components participating in a wide variety of cognitive processes? Studies have clearly established particular areas in the brain for processing human faces, the fusiform face area (FFA),[43] whereas other studies have compellingly argued that the FFA is actually a flexible area for visual processing automatized by expertise, which can be activated by cars in car experts, birds in bird experts, and Greebles (a novel variable stimuli) in trained Greeble experts.[44] In Gauthier's model, faces just happen to be the most universal area of expertise shared by most humans, but not all humans, as demonstrated by studies of autism.[45] Neuroimaging also emphasizes functional localization in space over transient functional neural networks in time. The brain's use of time and time-based coding schemes are essential components in understanding mechanisms of the mind, and the brain's ability to bind incoming multisensory information depends critically on the temporal window of integration.[46,47]

Despite the caveats aforementioned, neuroimaging (and previous neuroscience techniques, including electrophysiology and neuroanatomic dissection) has provided a wealth of data relevant to potential biologic mechanisms for psychodynamic models of the mind. Key regions include the amygdala, hippocampus, ventromedial prefrontal cortex, orbitofrontal cortex, dorsolateral prefrontal cortex, cingulate gyrus, and insula (**Table 1**).

SOME BRAIN REGIONS OF INTEREST FOR PSYCHOTHERAPY

Every region in the human brain has relevance for mental processes, and therefore for psychotherapy (**Table 2**). Following are descriptions of some key regions of special interest for affective and higher-order mental functions, such as fear conditioning, affective valence, emotional regulation, motivation, reward, memory, prediction, behavioral inhibition/response control, and mentalizing.

The amygdala, hippocampus, and medial prefrontal cortex (mPFC) have a high degree of connectivity with each other (and with other limbic, subcortical and neocortical regions), and an integrative role at the interface of sensory, cognitive, affective, and behavioral processing.[48,49] Research indicates that the amygdala is necessary for ascribing an affective valence to stimuli and for the stress/fear response and conditioning; the hippocampus is necessary for proper contextual control of this response and for declarative memory functions; and the mPFC exerts inhibitory/modulatory control over the response.[50] Although the hippocampus has traditionally been studied in relation to retrieving memories about the past, recent work suggests that the hippocampal system may be better understood as facilitating predictions about upcoming events.[51] Functional imaging and clinical lesion research has shown that key aspects of the neural circuits of fear discovered through animal studies are relevant to human fear.[52–55]

In addition to considering brain regions with distinct functions, gradients, from ventral/medial to dorsal/lateral and from subcortical/limbic to neocortical, are central to current models of emotional processing and regulation. Gradients coordinate processes ranging from detection of emotional salience and valence; to neuroendocrine, somatic, and autonomic responses; to conflict detection and response selection; to higher-order goal-directed behavioral responses; to conscious/effortful modulation and control.[48,56–58]

AMYGDALA

Research in animals on fear conditioning has implicated circuits centered around the amygdala in the acquisition, storage, expression, and extinction of fear memory.[59–61]

Table 1
Neuroimaging studies of psychotherapy effects on brain function

Article	Diagnosis	Therapy	Imaging Tool	ROI: Changes With Treatment
Baxter et al,[205] 1992	OCD	CBT: exposure	PET	Caudate nucleus (R >L) (decreased blood flow)
Beutel et al,[167] 2010	Panic disorder	PDPT	fMRI	Amygdala and hippocampus (decreased), prefrontal (increased)
Bor et al,[206] 2011	Schizophrenia	CRT	fMRI	L inferior/middle frontal and cingulate gyri, inferior parietal lobule (increases to spatial task)
Brody et al,[207] 2001	MDD severe	IPT	PET	Prefrontal and lower temporal regions (normalized higher metabolism in MDD)
de Greck et al,[168] 2011	Somatoform disorder	PDPT	fMRI	L postcentral gyrus, R ventroposterior thalamus (normalization of differentiation of rewarding events)
de Lange et al,[208] 2008	Chronic fatigue syndrome	CBT	MRI	Lateral prefrontal cortex increases in gray matter volume (reversed cerebral atrophy)
Furmark et al,[209] 2002	Social phobia	CBT	PET	Amygdala, hippocampus, adjacent cortex (decreased blood flow, proportional to improvement)
Goldin & Gross,[210] 2010	Social phobia	MBSR	fMRI	Amygdala (decrease)
Goossens et al,[211] 2007	Specific phobia	CBT: exposure	fMRI	Amygdala, anterior cingulate, and insula (activity decreased from elevated baseline)
Haut et al,[212] 2010	Schizophrenia	CRT: memory-focused	fMRI	Dorsolateral prefrontal, anterior cingulate, and frontopolar cortex (increased)
Hoekzema et al,[213] 2010	ADHD	Cognitive training	fMRI	Orbitofrontal, superior frontal, middle temporal, inferior frontal, cerebellar (increased)
Huyser et al,[214] 2010	OCD (pediatric)	CBT	fMRI	Dorsolateral prefrontal and parietal (increased, normalized)
Kennedy et al,[215] 2007	MDD	CBT	PET	Orbitofrontal and L dorsomedial prefrontal, posterior cingulate (decreased); R occipital-temporal, L temporal, and subgenual cingulate (increased)

Kumari et al,[216] 2011	Psychosis	CBT: cognitive	fMRI	Inferior frontal, insula, thalamus, putamen, occipital (decreases to negative stimuli)
Lindauer et al,[217] 2008	PTSD	Eclectic psycho-therapy	SPECT	R middle frontal gyrus (decreased)
Martin et al,[218] 2001	MDD	IPT	SPECT	R basal ganglia and R posterior cingulate gyrus (increased activation)
Nakatani et al,[219] 2003	OCD	CBT: exposure	SPECT (Xenon)	R caudate (decreased blood flow from elevated in baseline OCD)
Prasko et al,[220] 2004	Panic disorder	CBT	PET	R inferior temporal gyrus, R superior and inferior frontal gyri (decreases); L inferior frontal gyrus, L middle temporal gyrus, and L insula (increases)
Ritchey et al,[171] 2011	MDD	CBT	fMRI	Ventromedial prefrontal (increased); amygdala, caudate, hippocampus (enhanced arousal responses); anterior temporal (reversal of valence effects)
Sakai et al,[221] 2006	Panic disorder	CBT	PET	R hippocampus, L anterior cingulate, L cerebellum, pons (decreased); medial prefrontal (increased)
Saxena et al,[222] 2009	OCD	CBT: exposure (brief)	PET	Thalamus (bilateral decreases) R dorsal anterior cingulate (increase)
Schwartz et al,[223] 1996	OCD	CBT: exposure	PET	Caudate nucleus (R > L) (decreased blood flow)
Vollstädt-Klein et al,[224] 2011	Alcohol-dependent	CET	fMRI	L ventral striatum (decreased)
Vocks et al,[225] 2011	Anorexia and bulimia	CBT: body image therapy	fMRI	L middle temporal gyrus (extrastriate body area), bilateral middle frontal gyri
Yamanishi et al,[226] 2009	OCD	CBT: exposure	SPECT	L medial prefrontal, bilateral middle frontal gyri (decreased)

Abbreviations: ADHD, attention deficit hyperactivity disorder; CBT, cognitive behavior therapy; CET, cue-exposure–based extinction training; CRT, cognitive remediation therapy; fMRI, functional MRI; IPT, interpersonal therapy; L, left; MBSR, mindfulness-based stress reduction; MDD, major depressive disorder; OCD, obsessive compulsive disorder; PDPT, psychodynamic psychotherapy; PET, Positron emission tomography; PTSD, Posttraumatic stress disorder; R, right; ROI, regions of interest (localized brain areas affected by psychotherapy); SPECT, single-photon emission computed tomography.

Table 2
Summary of key regions, their proposed functions, findings implicating them in psychopathology, and relevant psychoanalytic concepts[a]

Region of Interest	Function	Psychiatric Pathology	Psychodynamic Concepts of Relevance
Amygdala	Negative emotional processing, fear conditioning, emotional memory, emotional expression, emotional evaluation, motivated behavior	Hyperactive in depression,[227,228] hyperactive to traumatic stimuli in posttraumatic stress disorder, impaired emotional memory after damage	Id, drives, pleasure-unpleasure principal
Brainstem ascending neurotransmitter nuclei	Neuromodulation of motivational, attentional, and emotional processing, generalized arousal and activational functions	Associated with autonomic dysfunction in panic/anxiety disorder[229,230]	Psychic energy, drives
Dorsal anterior cingulate	Cognitive functions: modulation of attention or executive functions, response selection, monitoring competition, motivation, error detection, working memory, task demand anticipation	Hypoactive in depression,[231,232] increases in activity, accompany successful treatment of depression with cognitive behavioral therapy[176]	Ego, superego, top-down selection of schema
Dorsomedial prefrontal cortex	Top-down cognitive processing of complex fear signals, cognitive interpretation of emotional stimuli, cognitive regulation of emotion, attention to emotional experience, mentalizing (attending to the mental states of self or others)	Hypoactive in depression[231,232]	Ego, superego, schemas object relations
Dorsolateral prefrontal cortex	Working memory, attention, executive cognitive functions, effortful control (degree of difficulty), emotion/cognition interactions in negative mood	Hypoactive in depression[231–233]	Ego, superego
Hippocampus: posterior/dorsal (spatial/navigational) anterior/ventral (emotional)	Declarative memory, relational processing, emotional memory, contextual control of fear	Hypoactive in geriatric depression,[234] decreased volume with depression,[235] Animal literature shows decreased spine-density premenstrually[236]	Schemas, ego, object relations (anterior/ventral: id)
Insula	Visceral arousal, mediating subjective feeling states, interoceptive tasks, transient skin conductance responses	Hyperactive in depression[237,238]	Id, pleasure-unpleasure principal

Lateral orbitofrontal cortex	Multimodal sensory processing/evaluation, emotional valence, emotional salience, motivation, unpleasantness/punishment, socioemotional control	Hyperactive to emotional stimuli in depression,[233,239] abnormal cytoarchitecture in depression,[240] inverse relationship between metabolism and depression severity[227]	Superego, ego, pleasure-unpleasure principal
Medial orbitofrontal cortex	Visceromotor link, modulation of arousal and behavior, emotional valence, emotional salience, motivation, pleasantness/reward socioemotional control	Behavioral disinhibition, "acquired sociopath" syndrome after damage, impulse dyscontrol	Superego, ego, pleasure-unpleasure principal
Middle/posterior cingulate	Integration of sensory signals, connection between sensory and limbic areas	Hyperactive in depression[237,238]	Ego
Rostral anterior cingulate	Transition zone that may help to orchestrate the reciprocal relationship between the subgenual (emotional) and dorsal (cognitive) subdivisions anterior cingulate	Differentiates treatment responders (hypermetabolism) from nonresponders (hypometabolism) in depression[175,241]	Ego
Subgenual cingulate	Affective functions: assesses the salience of emotional and motivational information and regulates emotional responses	Hypoactive in depression,[237,242] decreased volume in depression[243,244]	Pleasure-unpleasure principal
Superior temporal sulcus	Multimodal sensory convergence zone, complex behavior, proposed to be concerned with the sensory signals that elicit mentalizing	Hyperactivity for negative affect disturbances in depression,[245] increased volume in depression[246]	Schemas, object relations, ego, superego
Thalamus/striatum	Subcortical nuclei involved in circuits/loops coordinating behavior with discrete subregions and pathways mediating specific behavioral/emotional/perceptual/cognitive functions, oscillating circuitry	Hyperactive left medial thalamus[227] and hypoactive caudate in depression[227,247]	Unconscious/nonconscious processing
Ventral striatum	Positive (hedonic) emotional processing, selection of motivated behavioral responses, reward/motivation, addiction	Failure of ventral striatal activation to positive stimuli in depression (Epstein, personal communication, 2005), substance abuse	Pleasure-unpleasure, principal wishes, drives

[a] This table is necessarily selective, and markedly condenses the available information on these regions, representing functions and dysfunctions thought to be of particular relevance. The "psychoanalytic concept of relevance" is highly speculative and meant to stimulate discussion rather than propose fact.

Within the amygdala, sensory information enters the lateral nucleus,[62] the plasticity underlying pavlovian fear conditioning occurs in the basolateral nucleus,[63] and outflow projections come from the central nucleus, which connects to a variety of hypothalamic and brain stem areas, mediating amygdalar output to behavioral, autonomic, and endocrine emotional response control systems.[64] In addition to encoding the emotional component of the memories formed during fear conditioning,[63–65] the amygdala also modulates the consolidation of memories formed in other brain regions.[66,67] Lesion analysis, electrophysiologic, and neuroimaging studies have demonstrated that the amygdala is important for responsivity to affective stimuli; the acquisition and expression of emotional/arousing memories; and the ability to recognize emotion in human faces.[52,66,68,69]

VENTRAL STRIATUM

The amygdala is responsive to reward and aversive stimuli.[70–72] The ventral, or limbic, striatum (and particularly the nucleus accumbens) is interconnected with the amygdala, hippocampus, and mPFC, and plays a key role in integrating relevant motivational information in the context of goal-directed behavior[73,74] and is a central node in reward circuitry. Neuroimaging has demonstrated a failure of ventral striatal activation to positive stimuli in patients with depression, compared with normal control subjects, and in patients with PMDD.[75]

HIPPOCAMPUS

The hippocampus has been implicated in the contextual control of fear through interactions with the amygdala.[59,76–78] Within the hippocampus, the entorhinal region is the way station for highly processed sensory information; the subiculum is the site of efferent output; and internal regions, such as the dentate gyrus (with mossy fiber projections) to CA3, may be most vulnerable to the effects of fear or stress. The afferent and efferent connectivity of the hippocampus changes moving from the posterior/dorsal (septal) to the anterior/ventral (temporal) pole.[79] Lesion and electrophysiologic studies indicate that the posterior/dorsal hippocampal formation is more important for spatial learning,[80,81] whereas the anterior/ventral hippocampus is necessary for unconditioned fear.[82] More "visceral" regions, such as the amygdala and caudal piriform cortex, send information through the rostromedial entorhinal cortex to the anterior/temporal (ventral) one-third of the hippocampus.[83–86] A growing body of data implicates the anterior/ventral hippocampus in regulation of the hypothalamic-pituitary-adrenal axis and modulation of mesocorticolimbic dopaminergic function.[87–92] The anterior hippocampus (of the human) has been implicated in the pathogenesis of schizophrenia, and neonatal damage to the corresponding ventral hippocampus of the rodent is an intriguing animal model of schizophrenia.[93–107]

FUSIFORM GYRUS

The fusiform gyrus processes visual properties of objects.[108] Images of humans and animals differentially activate the lateral portion of the fusiform gyrus,[43,109,110] whereas manipulable objects (tools and utensils) differentially activate the medial fusiform gyrus.[111] Highly contextualized stimuli, such as houses and scenes, activate the parahippocampal gyrus.[112] Again, the FFA can be activated by cars in car experts, birds in bird experts, and Greebles in Greeble experts. Further work is required to refine the understanding of how these object category–specific subdivisions of the fusiform area are formed, and to what extent these subdivisions are based on physical properties of objects (bottom-up from sensory cortex), abstract concepts (top-down from prefrontal cortex), or other network properties related to how representations of these objects are stored in the brain. Although the fusiform gyrus is part of the ventral stream (visual object recognition), evidence shows that neural specificity for objects in the fusiform gyrus is determined partly by similarity metrics computed over information that is stored elsewhere.[113] For example, neural specificity for animals, faces, objects, or places may depend on dorsal stream regions mediating object-directed action,[113] or could conceivably depend on multimodal sensory information or abstract concepts.

mPFC

The mPFC has been implicated in the regulation of fear by changes in environmental circumstances through interactions with the amygdala.[114,115] Several distinct areas in the human mPFC are of interest. The ventral anterior cingulate cortex is most analogous to the region implicated by Ledoux and Muller[50] in the rodent model; has strong connections with the amygdala, periaqueductal gray, nucleus accumbens, hypothalamus, anterior insula, hippocampus, and orbitofrontal cortex[116]; and is highly involved in emotional/motivational (rather than more dorsally located cognitive or motor) regulation.[116] It has been proposed to assess the salience of emotional and motivational information and to regulate emotional responses.[116–119] The dorsal anterior cingulate cortex has strong reciprocal connections with the lateral prefrontal cortex, parietal cortex, premotor cortex, and supplementary motor cortex,[116] and has been proposed to modulate attention or executive functions through influencing response selection, monitoring competition, motivation, error detection, working memory, and task demand anticipation.[116–123] The medial orbitofrontal cortex (OFC) receives projections from the lateral amygdalar nuclei and projects to the central nucleus, and is in a position to modulate amygdala output based on changing contingencies.

REGIONS ASSOCIATED WITH RESPONSE INHIBITION

Prepotent response inhibition is at least partly mediated by the prefrontal cortex (PFC).[124] For example, OFC dysfunction has long been associated with behavioral disinhibition.[125] An "acquired sociopathic" syndrome has been described after ventromedial PFC damage,[125] prompting the hypothesis that impaired ventromedial PFC function contributes to impulse dyscontrol in antisocial personality disorder.[126]

The go/no-go task has been adapted in many variations to probe response inhibition. Go/no-go tasks involve execution or inhibition of a prepotent motor response, triggered by a go- or no-go stimulus, respectively. Demand to respond quickly creates a prepotent response tone, which must be inhibited when cued by a no-go stimulus. Although seemingly behaviorally simple, the task involves cognitive and motor subprocesses, including stimulus discrimination, response selection, motor preparation, response inhibition, and error monitoring. Thus, go/no-go deficits can be attributed to several potential component process impairments. Frontal regions variably implicated in prepotent motor response suppression include OFC,[127,128] dorsolateral PFC,[127–131] middle PFC,[131,132] inferior PFC,[130,132,133] anterior cingulate cortex,[130,134] supplementary motor area,[131,135] and presupplementary motor area.[136] Nonfrontal regions have also been implicated, including parietal,[131,132,135] temporal,[128,131,132] and occipital.[131]

Many psychiatric disorders involve behavioral inhibitory failure,[137] which often becomes prominent within certain emotional contexts.[138] Inconsistencies of activation patterns observed across response inhibition studies have prompted some investigators to consider a multidomain model of inhibitory control,[139] in which different functions (eg, motor vs cognitive) are at least partly regulated by different inhibitory mechanisms, correspondingly mediated by different brain regions. Accordingly, brain activation patterns associated with inhibitory control partly depend on the specific cognitive/behavioral domain needing to be inhibited, and therefore the type of inhibitory processes invoked.[139]

REGIONS ASSOCIATED WITH MENTALIZING

Mentalizing (theory of mind) allows one to attend to the desires, attitudes, and beliefs of the self and others. The mentalizing system of the brain is thought to allow implicit attribution of intentions and other mental states starting around 18 months of age, and to allow explicit mentalizing between the ages of 4 and 6 years.[140] Neuroimaging studies of mentalizing in human adults have consistently found activation in the dorsomedial PFC (specifically the anterior part of the paracingulate cortex, anterior to the genu of the corpus callosum and the anterior cingulate cortex proper), the temporal poles, and the posterior superior temporal sulcus (STS).[140]

Neuroimaging studies of mentalizing have used a wide range of tasks, including stories in which behavior is dependent on protagonist intentions or false belief,[141–143] cartoon strips only interpretable in terms of protagonist intentions or false beliefs,[142–144] decisions requiring the subject to infer something about the knowledge and beliefs of someone who lived 500 years ago,[145] stories involving social transgressions,[146] and attributions of mental states to the movement of abstract shapes.[147,148]

There is evidence that the STS is concerned with the nature of the sensory signals that elicit mentalizing.[140] Studies of STS neuroanatomical connectivity demonstrate that it a multimodal sensory convergence zone with connections to the limbic system.[149] Neuroimaging studies show STS activation for biologic motion,[150–152] integration of auditory and visual (moving mouths) speech,[153,154] images of faces and animals,[111] and semantic decisions about living things. The STS seems to supply knowledge about and prediction of complex behavior, representing some of the key information required for mentalizing.[140]

Neuroimaging studies during game playing found activity in the dorsomedial PFC (and only in the dorsomedial PFC) when the volunteers believed that they were interacting with another person, but not when they believed they were interacting with a computer,[155,156] indicating that dorsomedial PFC activity reflects the attitude taken toward the sensory signals that elicit mentalizing. Dorsomedial PFC has been associated with top-down cognitive processing of complex fear signals. Increased activity in this region correlated with decreased skin conductance response frequency during exposure to fearful faces.[157] Activity in this region also increased, whereas activity in the insula and amygdala decreased, during cognitive interpretation of emotional stimuli (compared with passive viewing of this stimuli).[158] Cognitive regulation of emotion has been associated with this region in fMRI studies of emotional reappraisal.[159] Attention to emotional experience (compared with passive experience) has also been found to increase activity in the dorsomedial PFC.[160,161] A similar distinction is found in a study of pain wherein the mental attitude toward pain (as opposed to the physical pain stimulus) is represented in the dorsomedial PFC.[162] Thus, this region of the dorsomedial PFC seems to be engaged when attending to the mental states of self or others.[140,163]

PSYCHOTHERAPY CHANGES THE BRAIN

Increasing neuroimaging literature shows measurable changes in brain function after psychotherapeutic intervention[164,165] (see **Table 1**). For example, behavioral therapy for anxiety disorders has been associated with attenuation of neuroimaging abnormalities in regions associated with the pathophysiology of anxiety.[166] Most of these studies to date focus on time-limited evidence-based therapies (cognitive behavior therapy [CBT], interpersonal psychotherapy). Only a few studies to date have examined neuroimaging before and after psychodynamic psychotherapy. A study of patients with panic disorder (compared with normal controls) found normalization of initially high limbic (hippocampus and amygdala) and low prefrontal activation to negative words after short-term psychodynamic inpatient treatment.[167] A study of patients with somatoform disorder showed diminished differentiation between rewarding and nonrewarding events in regions involved in sensory processing, which normalized after multimodal psychodynamic psychotherapy.[168]

Manualized psychoanalytic psychotherapy tested in randomized control trials (such as Milrod's psychodynamic therapy for panic disorder) should lead to further neuroimaging studies of psychodynamic psychotherapy in the near future. A recent review of randomized controlled trials of psychodynamic psychotherapy applied the Randomized Controlled Trial Psychotherapy Quality Rating Scale (RCT-PQRS) to 94 randomized controlled trials of psychodynamic psychotherapy published between 1974 and May 2010.[169] This study concluded that existing randomized controlled trials of psychodynamic psychotherapy are promising but mostly show superiority of psychodynamic psychotherapy to an inactive comparator, and further randomized controlled trials of adequate quality and sample size are needed to replicate findings of existing positive trials for specific disorders.

NEUROIMAGING TO PREDICT TREATMENT OUTCOME

Patient selection is one of the most difficult problems in psychotherapeutic treatment. Currently no reliable and valid methods exist to determine which patients will respond best to psychodynamic psychotherapy versus CBT versus medication, or a combination of these interventions. The length of treatment required for symptom remission is also difficult to anticipate, because it varies from case to case. One of the desired clinical uses of neuroimaging is to identify biomarkers that can be used to predict treatment response. Although this is not yet part clinical practice, a growing number of studies are showing that neuroimaging has the potential to be used in this way.

Major Depressive Disorder

A study of major depressive disorder (MDD) has shown that pretreatment OFC functional connectivity levels as measured with fMRI may be a useful marker for therapy response to mirtazapine and venlafaxine.[170] Another MDD study showed that CBT-related symptom improvement was predicted by increased baseline activity in ventromedial PFC and by valence effects in the anterior temporal lobe and dorsolateral PFC.[171] A study of adolescent MDD showed that pretreatment reward–related brain activity in the striatum and medial PFC was related to response to treatment by CBT alone and CBT in combination with a selective serotonin reuptake inhibitor.[172] A SPECT study of MDD showed that pretreatment hypermetabolism at the interface of the pregenual and subgenual cingulate cortices predicted which patients would not experience a response to CBT or venlafaxine.[173] A previous study similarly reported relative hypoactivity in the ventral anterior cingulate cortex, and amygdala hyperactivity in patients with depression responsive to treatment with CBT.[174] However, a PET study of patients with depression showed that rostral anterior cingulate hypometabolism characterized those who would not experience a response to antidepressant drugs.[175] Distinct changes in frontal and limbic cortex seen with CBT relative to antidepressants (eg, paroxetine) may reflect modality-specific effects, implicating different mechanisms of action for improvement with psychotherapy as opposed to medication.[176] Helen Mayberg,[56] whose laboratory is responsible for most of the neuroimaging findings predicting treatment response in depression, has hypothesized that "limbic-cortical network" dysfunction combined with active intrinsic compensatory processes explains the heterogeneity of depressive symptoms observed clinically, and variations in pretreatment scan patterns described experimentally. She considers the synchronized modulation of these dysfunctional limbic-cortical pathways to be critical for illness remission, regardless of treatment modality.

Schizophrenia

A study of CBT in schizophrenia showed that stronger dorsolateral PFC activity and dorsolateral PFC–cerebellum connectivity during a memory task at baseline was associated with clinical improvement in response to CBT for psychosis.[177] Multivariate neuroanatomic pattern classification on structural MRI data from individuals with a high risk of developing psychosis and healthy controls showed that this technique may reliably identify those at greatest risk for transition to psychosis.[178]

Neuroimaging Combined With Genetics

In addition to baseline neuroimaging as a potential predictor of treatment outcomes, genetics and molecular markers in combination with neuroimaging findings is a potentially powerful tool for predicting treatment response.

SCHEMAS

Schemas, implicit preexisting knowledge structures or associative networks, are thought to allow for efficient interpretation of new sensory input and rapid selection of behavioral and affective responses.[179–181] Schemas are crucial for psychoanalysis, wherein a significant part of the therapeutic process is the activation of implicitly learned relations and expectations to make them accessible to the analyst for change. Schemas are difficult to study empirically because they are implicit (not accessible to self-report) and idiosyncratic (based on individual experiences).

However, a growing body of literature implicates the hippocampus in gradual incorporation of novel information into long-term memory through binding, reactivating, and strengthening distributed cortical–cortical connections and the ventromedial prefrontal cortex as a central node in these representational networks over time.[182] Studies also suggest that the PFC and temporal cortex play central roles in integrating multiple information sources in processing concepts.[183–186]

Conceptual Processing Linked With Perceptual Processing

A key concept when considering the neurobiologic mechanism of schemas is that conceptual processing is tied to perceptual processing.[187] Object recognition, attitude, and social perception are tied to embodiment and are severely inhibited when embodiment is prohibited.[188] For example, individuals who lack one of the sensory modalities early in development (eg, blindness or deafness) have been shown to organize schemas differently at the neural level because the missing modality cannot play the same role in schema formation.[189] According to this theory, schemas (which are likely no different from what is generally meant by "concepts," or thoughts that are not based in just one sensory modality, such as "car," "justice," or "mother") arise through the establishment of convergent cross-modal (ie, multisensory) associations related to a perception or action.[190] Thus, cross-modal conceptual areas (such as those in the midtemporal cortex, Wernicke area, the hippocampal–entorhinal complex, and posterior parietal cortex) serve as organizing hubs for representations of objects, people, or events. For example, popcorn may be imagined purely visually, but a more complete representation includes links to all the other sensory input relevant for a particular individual (eg, the sound of popping, the smell of melted butter, or even the sound of people whispering in the dark, the smell of an old movie theater). In other words, every meaningful concept is stored in a multisensory way. The mental representation fluctuates according to what is called for by selective attention. The more concretely physical and basic the task (eg, "how do I pick up this piece of popcorn?), the more narrow its tuning.[184] Therefore, these basic parts have very precise tuning (eg, retinotopic images, individual pitches), whereas their controlling hubs have broader tuning and represent more complex and abstract entities.

Concept of "Priming"

Cognitive scientists have developed clever paradigms for investigating the nature of object representations from perceptual to conceptual levels in an unbiased data-driven manner.[184] These paradigms use the concept of "priming"; that is, exposing a person to a particular stimulus or concept before the actual task, thereby increasing the speed and accuracy with which the task is performed. Multiple repetitions of the same visual stimulus lead to large temporary decreases in neural activity throughout the visual brain in cells that are responsive to the stimulus. This technique has been used to establish separate sites within prefrontal cortex representing broad and narrow conceptual tuning, and the representation of broad conceptual information, and form sensitive information, in the temporal cortex and as early as the extrastriate cortex.[184]

Using experimental data derived from this approach, a theoretical model has been proposed to explain the role of different brain structures in schema processing. The hippocampus is critical for binding, reactivating, and strengthening distributed cortical–cortical connections. The prefrontal cortex is a central node in storing the information necessary for selecting representational networks when they are needed. Bottom-up activation of representations through evocative sensory experiences can also occur. Divergent sensory areas are not merely activated in parallel through hippocampal or prefrontal connections, but are also influenced by each other; for example, recognition of a "tool" in the visual cortex influences which components of the motor cortex are most likely to activate, and vice versa.[113]

Schemas for Social Concepts

Schemas for social concepts depend on activity in specific neural networks.[185] Deficits in social schemas have implications for social functioning. For example, rigid adherence to a negative schema may result in an individual having a negative reaction to a positive event. Neurobiologic studies in humans and nonhuman primates suggest that the temporal cortex (particularly anteriorly) plays a central role in integrating multiple information sources in the processing of socially and emotionally relevant concepts.[183,186] A validated behavioral task (in which participants display implicit biases in their memory, affect, and behavior based on the resemblance between a new "stranger" and a significant person in their lives) allowed Andersen and colleagues[191,192] to study the influence of an individual's social schemas (compared with those supplied by another participant or a random assortment of the participant's own words). This task is perfectly suited to studying the neurobiology of implicit schemas with fMRI in which clear experimental control conditions are essential.[193]

AUTISM AND SCHEMAS

Evidence suggests that individuals with autism spectrum disorders (ASD) have deficits in their ability to form and use schemas.[194,195] A deficit in the use of schemas in ASD is consistent with another finding, first described by Frith,[196] that individuals with ASD have "weak central coherence" or a tendency toward processing local, or detail-oriented, sensory information over global or integrated impressions.[197,198] Neuropsychological studies have indicated differential hemisphere dominance for global (right) or local (left) aspects of complex visual scenes, but evidence indicates that these relative differential hemispheric activations during global and local processing may be modified by stimulus category.[199] Studies that measured the relative preference for local versus global perception in individuals with high-functioning ASD using established behavioral measures (subjects are shown pictures of large letters composed of smaller letters[200] or must locate small shapes within more complicated ones[201]) have reported normal levels of overall accuracy in global processing, yet increased reaction time and attentional demands.[202,203] Thus, high-functioning individuals with ASD may develop compensatory strategies for applying schemas, but these strategies may be less efficient than those used by healthy individuals. It is interesting to hypothesize how "strong central coherence" or a tendency toward processing global or integrated impressions over local or detail-oriented sensory information may be reflected in psychopathology. One small study showed an abnormal global processing advantage in a global–local task in schizotypal personality disorder compared with controls.[204]

SUMMARY

Cognitive science, molecular biology, genetics, and neuroimaging offer ever increasing insight into brain function. Statistical methods in fMRI are complex, and interpreting tantalizing images of neural activity without understanding these limitations is problematic. Interpreting the results from neuroimaging paradigms is rarely straightforward, and requires constantly challenging assumptions about the mechanisms of the mind. Is the mind composed of highly specialized components for specific aspects of cognition, or more general-purpose components participating in a wide variety of cognitive processes? More data inevitably lead to more questions. Individual variability is a central problem in neuroscience research. Psychodynamic clinicians and theorists have an important role to play in ensuring that the most clinically relevant and interesting questions are being asked. A dynamic perspective can assist researchers by helping them avoid oversimplifying human emotional or cognitive processes, and recognize how their own biases affect the questions they ask and data interpretation.

This article addressed only a fraction of the neuroscience studies relevant to psychodynamic models and interventions. Genetics, molecular biology, and neuroimaging may provide insight into the neurobiologic bases of individual psychological differences and treatment response in patients. A greater understanding of the brain regions involved in emotional processing (amygdala), memory formation and future prediction (hippocampus), and top-down regulation (prefrontal cortex) is essential for the continuing refinement of models of the mind. Schemas are of great interest for psychodynamic work, and neuroscience is beginning to elucidate how the hippocampus, multimodal association areas, primary sensory areas, and prefrontal cortex work together to store, reactivate, change, and make use of schemas dynamically over time. It is also interesting to hypothesize how "strong central coherence" or a tendency toward processing global or integrated impressions over local or detail-oriented sensory information (the opposite situation to that seen in ASD) may be reflected in psychopathology. The combined efforts of neuroscientists studying the brain and psychodynamic clinicians and theorists studying the mind are needed to unravel the mechanisms of human mental functioning.

REFERENCES

1. Blass RB, Carmeli Z. The case against neuropsychoanalysis. On fallacies underlying psychoanalysis' latest scientific trend and its negative impact on psychoanalytic discourse. Int J Psychoanal 2007;88(Pt 1):19–40.
2. Breger L. Psychoanalysis is not science. Humanities working paper 6. Pasadena (CA): California Institute of Technology; 1978.
3. Edelson M. Hypothesis and evidence in psychoanalysis. Chicago: University of Chicago Press; 1984.
4. Kandel ER. Biology and the future of psychoanalysis: a new intellectual framework for psychiatry revisited. Am J Psychiatry 1999;156(4):505–24.
5. Kernberg O. Psychoanalytic affect theory in the light of contemporary neurobiological findings. In: The Inseparable Nature of Love and Aggression. Washington, DC: American Psychiatric Press; 2012. p. 183–200.
6. Albright TD, Jessell TM, Kandel ER, et al. Neural science: a century of progress and the mysteries that remain. Cell 2000;25(Suppl 100):S1–55.
7. Tyson P, Tyson RL. Psychoanalytic theories of development: an integration. New Haven (CT): Yale University Press; 1990.
8. Fonagy P, Target M, Steele M, et al. Psychoanalytic perspectives on developmental psychopathology. In: Cicchetti D, Cohen DJ, editors. Developmental psychopathology. New York: John Wiley & Sons; 1995. p. 504–54
9. Sroufe LA, Rutter M. The domain of developmental psychopathology. Child Dev 1984;55(1):17–29.
10. Beutel ME, Stern E, Silbersweig DA. The emerging dialogue between psychoanalysis and neuroscience: neuroimaging perspectives. J Am Psychoanal Assoc 2003;51(3):773–801.
11. Andreasen NC. Linking mind and brain in the study of mental illnesses: a project for a scientific psychopathology. Science 1997;275(5306):1586–93.
12. Cooper AM. Will neurobiology influence psychoanalysis? Am J Psychiatry 1985; 142(12):1395–402.
13. Gabbard GO. A neurobiologically informed perspective on psychotherapy. Br J Psychiatry 2000;177:117–22.
14. Bennett CM, Baird AA, Miller MB, et al. Neural correlates of interspecies perspective taking in the post-mortem atlantic salmon: an argument for proper multiple comparisons correction. Journal of Serendipitous and Unexpected Results 2010;1(1):1–5.
15. Protopopescu X, Tuescher O, Pan H, et al. Toward a functional neuroanatomy of premenstrual dysphoric disorder. J Affect Disord 2008;108(1–2):87–94.
16. Greenspan RJ. The flexible genome. Nat Rev Genet 2001;2(5):383–7.
17. Chouard T, Darwin. 200: beneath the surface. Nature 2008;456(7220):300–3.
18. Goaillard JM, Taylor AL, Schulz DJ, et al. Functional consequences of animal-to-animal variation in circuit parameters. Nat Neurosci 2009;12(11):1424–30.
19. Akhtar S. Happiness: origins, forms, and technical relevance. Am J Psychoanal 2010;70(3):219–44.
20. Freud S. The resistances to psycho-analysis. In: Strachey J, editor. The standard edition of the complete psychological works of Sigmund Freud, volume XIX (1923–1925): the ego and the id and other works. London: Hogarth; 1925.

21. Franklin TB, Mansuy IM. Epigenetic inheritance in mammals: evidence for the impact of adverse environmental effects. Neurobiol Dis 2010;39(1):61–5.
22. Chen ZY, Jing D, Bath KG, et al. Genetic variant BDNF (Val66Met) polymorphism alters anxiety-related behavior. Science 2006;314(5796):140–3.
23. Yu H, Wang Y, Pattwell S, et al. Variant BDNF Val66Met polymorphism affects extinction of conditioned aversive memory. J Neurosci 2009;29(13):4056–64.
24. Ninan I, Bath KG, Dagar K, et al. The BDNF Val66Met polymorphism impairs NMDA receptor-dependent synaptic plasticity in the hippocampus. J Neurosci 2010;30(26):8866–70.
25. Bath KG, Jing DQ, Dincheva I, et al. BDNF Val66Met impairs fluoxetine-induced enhancement of adult hippocampus plasticity. Neuropsychopharmacology 2012;37(5):1297–304.
26. Spencer JL, Waters EM, Milner TA, et al. BDNF variant Val66Met interacts with estrous cycle in the control of hippocampal function. Proc Natl Acad Sci U S A 2010;107(9):4395–400.
27. Soliman F, Glatt CE, Bath KG, et al. A genetic variant BDNF polymorphism alters extinction learning in both mouse and human. Science 2010;327(5967):863–6.
28. Scharinger C, Rabl U, Pezawas L, et al. The genetic blueprint of major depressive disorder: contributions of imaging genetics studies. World J Biol Psychiatry 2011;12(7):474–88.
29. Bilder RM, Volavka J, Czobor P, et al. Neurocognitive correlates of the COMT Val(158)Met polymorphism in chronic schizophrenia. Biol Psychiatry 2002; 52(7):701–7.
30. Cohen H, Neumann L, Glazer Y, et al. The relationship between a common catechol-O-methyltransferase (COMT) polymorphism val(158) met and fibromyalgia. Clin Exp Rheumatol 2009;27(5 Suppl 56):S51–6.
31. Jensen KB, Lonsdorf TB, Schalling M, et al. Increased sensitivity to thermal pain following a single opiate dose is influenced by the COMT val(158)met polymorphism. PLoS One 2009;4(6):e6016.
32. Harris SE, Wright AF, Hayward C, et al. The functional COMT polymorphism, Val 158 Met, is associated with logical memory and the personality trait intellect/imagination in a cohort of healthy 79 year olds. Neurosci Lett 2005;385(1):1–6.
33. Wagner S, Baskaya O, Anicker NJ, et al. The catechol o-methyltransferase (COMT) val(158)met polymorphism modulates the association of serious life events (SLE) and impulsive aggression in female patients with borderline personality disorder (BPD). Acta Psychiatr Scand 2010;122(2):110–7.
34. Williams LM, Gatt JM, Grieve SM, et al. COMT Val(108/158)Met polymorphism effects on emotional brain function and negativity bias. Neuroimage 2010; 53(3):918–25.
35. Olsson CA, Byrnes GB, Anney RJ, et al. COMT Val(158)Met and 5HTTLPR functional loci interact to predict persistence of anxiety across adolescence: results from the Victorian adolescent health cohort study. Genes Brain Behav 2007;6(7): 647–52.
36. Markov V, Krug A, Krach S, et al. Genetic variation in schizophrenia-risk-gene dysbindin 1 modulates brain activation in anterior cingulate cortex and right temporal gyrus during language production in healthy individuals. Neuroimage 2009;47(4):2016–22.
37. Kircher T, Krug A, Markov V, et al. Genetic variation in the schizophrenia-risk gene neuregulin 1 correlates with brain activation and impaired speech production in a verbal fluency task in healthy individuals. Hum Brain Mapp 2009;30(10): 3406–16.

38. Bertolino A, Caforio G, Blasi G, et al. Interaction of COMT (Val(108/158)Met) genotype and olanzapine treatment on prefrontal cortical function in patients with schizophrenia. Am J Psychiatry 2004;161(10):1798–805.
39. Rebollo-Mesa I, Picchioni M, Shaikh M, et al. COMT (Val(158/108)Met) genotype moderates the impact of antipsychotic medication on verbal IQ in twins with schizophrenia. Psychiatr Genet 2011;21(2):98–105.
40. Frodl T, Möller HJ, Meisenzahl E. Neuroimaging genetics: new perspectives in research on major depression? Acta Psychiatr Scand 2008;118(5):363–72.
41. Klein TA, Neumann J, Reuter M, et al. Genetically determined differences in learning from errors. Science 2007;318(5856):1642–5.
42. Ekman P, Friesen WV. Pictures of facial affect. Palo Alto (CA): Consulting Psychologists Press; 1976.
43. Kanwisher N, McDermott J, Chun MM. The fusiform face area: a module in human extrastriate cortex specialized for face perception. J Neurosci 1997;17(11):4302–11.
44. Tarr MJ, Gauthier I. FFA: a flexible fusiform area for subordinate-level visual processing automatized by expertise. Nat Neurosci 2000;3(8):764–9.
45. Pierce K, Müller RA, Ambrose J, et al. Face processing occurs outside the fusiform 'face area' in autism: evidence from functional MRI. Brain 2001;124(Pt 10):2059–73.
46. Cohen MX. It's about time. Front Hum Neurosci 2011;5:2.
47. Powers AR, Hillock AR, Wallace MT. Perceptual training narrows the temporal window of multisensory binding. J Neurosci 2009;29(39):12265–74.
48. Mesulam M. Principles of behavioral neurology. In: Plum F, editor. Contemporary neurology. Philadelphia: F A David Company; 1985. p. 1–432.
49. Pandya DN, Yeterian EH. Architecture and connections of cortical association areas. In: Peters A, Jones EG, editors. Cerebral cortex, Association and Auditory Cortices, Vol. 4. New York: Plenum; 1984. p. 3–61.
50. Ledoux JE, Muller J. Emotional memory and psychopathology. Philos Trans R Soc Lond B Biol Sci 1997;352(1362):1719–26.
51. Buckner RL. The role of the hippocampus in prediction and imagination. Annu Rev Psychol 2010;61:27–48, C1.
52. Phelps EA, Anderson AK. Emotional memory: what does the amygdala do? Curr Biol 1997;7(5):R311 4.
53. Davidson RJ. Anxiety and affective style: role of prefrontal cortex and amygdala. Biol Psychiatry 2002;51(1):68–80.
54. Büchel C, Dolan RJ. Classical fear conditioning in functional neuroimaging. Curr Opin Neurobiol 2000;10(2):219–23.
55. Dolan RJ, Vuilleumier P. Amygdala automaticity in emotional processing. Ann N Y Acad Sci 2003;985:348–55.
56. Mayberg HS. Modulating dysfunctional limbic-cortical circuits in depression: towards development of brain-based algorithms for diagnosis and optimised treatment. Br Med Bull 2003;65:193–207.
57. Drevets WC. Neuroimaging and neuropathological studies of depression: implications for the cognitive-emotional features of mood disorders. Curr Opin Neurobiol 2001;11(2):240–9.
58. Phillips ML. Understanding the neurobiology of emotion perception: implications for psychiatry. Br J Psychiatry 2003;182:190–2.
59. Maren S. Auditory fear conditioning increases CS-elicited spike firing in lateral amygdala neurons even after extensive overtraining. Eur J Neurosci 2000;12(11):4047–54.

60. Fendt M, Fanselow MS. The neuroanatomical and neurochemical basis of conditioned fear. Neurosci Biobehav Rev 1999;23(5):743–60.
61. Davis M, Whalen PJ. The amygdala: vigilance and emotion. Mol Psychiatry 2001;6(1):13–34.
62. LeDoux JE, Cicchetti P, Xagoraris A, et al. The lateral amygdaloid nucleus: sensory interface of the amygdala in fear conditioning. J Neurosci 1990;10(4):1062–9.
63. Fanselow MS, LeDoux JE. Why we think plasticity underlying Pavlovian fear conditioning occurs in the basolateral amygdala. Neuron 1999;23(2):229–32.
64. Kandel E, Kandel ER, Schwartz J, et al. Principles of neural science. 4th edition. New York: McGraw-Hill Professional; 2000.
65. LeDoux J, LeDoux JE. The emotional brain. New York: Simon and Schuster; 1998.
66. Cahill L, Mcgaugh JL. The neurobiology of memory for emotional events: adrenergic activation and the amygdala. Proc West Pharmacol Soc 1996;39:81–4.
67. McGaugh JL, Cahill L, Roozendaal B. Involvement of the amygdala in memory storage: interaction with other brain systems. Proc Natl Acad Sci U S A 1996;93(24):13508–14.
68. LaBar KS, Gatenby JC, Gore JC, et al. Human amygdala activation during conditioned fear acquisition and extinction: a mixed-trial fMRI study. Neuron 1998;20(5):937–45.
69. Buchel C. Brain systems mediating aversive conditioning: an event-related fMRI study. Neuron 1998;20(5):947–57.
70. Everitt BJ, Morris KA, O'Brien A, et al. The basolateral amygdala-ventral striatal system and conditioned place preference: further evidence of limbic-striatal interactions underlying reward-related processes. Neuroscience 1991;42(1):1–8.
71. Everitt BJ, Parkinson JA, Olmstead MC, et al. Associative processes in addiction and reward. The role of amygdala-ventral striatal subsystems. Ann N Y Acad Sci 1999;877:412–38.
72. Cador M, Robbins TW, Everitt BJ. Involvement of the amygdala in stimulus-reward associations: interaction with the ventral striatum. Neuroscience 1989;30(1):77–86.
73. McGinty JF. Advancing from the ventral striatum to the extended amygdala. Implications for neuropsychiatry and drug abuse. Introduction. Ann N Y Acad Sci 1999;877:xii–xxv.
74. Heimer L, Alheid GF, de Olmos JS, et al. The accumbens: beyond the core-shell dichotomy. J Neuropsychiatry Clin Neurosci 1997;9(3):354–81.
75. Epstein J, Pan H, Kocsis JH, et al. Lack of ventral striatal response to positive stimuli in depressed versus normal subjects. Am J Psychiatry 2006;163(10):1784–90.
76. Kim JJ, Fanselow MS. Modality-specific retrograde amnesia of fear. Science 1992;256(5057):675–7.
77. Phillips RG, LeDoux JE. Differential contribution of amygdala and hippocampus to cued and contextual fear conditioning. Behav Neurosci 1992;106(2):274–85.
78. Frankland PW, Cestari V, Filipkowski RK, et al. The dorsal hippocampus is essential for context discrimination but not for contextual conditioning. Behav Neurosci 1998;112(4):863–74.
79. Moser MB, Moser EI. Functional differentiation in the hippocampus. Hippocampus 1998;8(6):608–19.
80. Moser MB, Moser EI, Forrest E, et al. Spatial learning with a minislab in the dorsal hippocampus. Proc Natl Acad Sci U S A 1995;92(21):9697–701.
81. Jung MW, Wiener SI, McNaughton BL. Comparison of spatial firing characteristics of units in dorsal and ventral hippocampus of the rat. J Neurosci 1994;14(12):7347–56.

82. Kjelstrup KG, Tuvnes FA, Steffenach HA, et al. Reduced fear expression after lesions of the ventral hippocampus. Proc Natl Acad Sci U S A 2002;99(16):10825–30.
83. Room P, Groenewegen HJ. Connections of the parahippocampal cortex in the cat. II. Subcortical afferents. J Comp Neurol 1986;251(4):451–73.
84. Room P, Groenewegen HJ. Connections of the parahippocampal cortex. I. Cortical afferents. J Comp Neurol 1986;251(4):415–50.
85. Insausti R, Amaral DG, Cowan WM. The entorhinal cortex of the monkey: III. Subcortical afferents. J Comp Neurol 1987;264(3):396–408.
86. Insausti R, Amaral DG, Cowan WM. The entorhinal cortex of the monkey: II. Cortical afferents. J Comp Neurol 1987;264(3):356–95.
87. Csernansky JG, Kerr S, Pruthi R, et al. Mesolimbic dopamine receptor increases two weeks following hippocampal kindling. Brain Res 1988;449(1–2):357–60.
88. Groenewegen HJ, Vermeulen-Van der Zee E, te Kortschot A, et al. Organization of the projections from the subiculum to the ventral striatum in the rat. A study using anterograde transport of phaseolus vulgaris leucoagglutinin. Neuroscience 1987;23(1):103–20.
89. Kelley AE, Domesick VB. The distribution of the projection from the hippocampal formation to the nucleus accumbens in the rat: an anterograde- and retrograde-horseradish peroxidase study. Neuroscience 1982;7(10):2321–35.
90. Lanier LP, Isaacson RL. Activity changes related to the location of lesion in the hippocampus. Behav Biol 1975;13(1):59–69.
91. Springer JE, Isaacson RL. Catecholamine alterations in basal ganglia after hippocampal lesions. Brain Res 1982;252(1):185–8.
92. Woodruff ML, Baisden RH, Fish BS. Forebrain catecholamine concentrations in the rat after neocortical and hippocampal lesions. Life Sci 1981;29(25):2603–7.
93. Bertolino A, Callicott JH, Elman I, et al. Regionally specific neuronal pathology in untreated patients with schizophrenia: a proton magnetic resonance spectroscopic imaging study. Biol Psychiatry 1998;43(9):641–8.
94. Bertolino A, Callicott JH, Nawroz S, et al. Reproducibility of proton magnetic resonance spectroscopic imaging in patients with schizophrenia. Neuropsychopharmacology 1998;18(1):1–9.
95. Bertolino A, Kumra S, Callicott JH, et al. Common pattern of cortical pathology in childhood-onset and adult-onset schizophrenia as identified by proton magnetic resonance spectroscopic imaging. Am J Psychiatry 1998;155(10):1376–83.
96. Bertolino A, Nawroz S, Mattay VS, et al. Regionally specific pattern of neurochemical pathology in schizophrenia as assessed by multislice proton magnetic resonance spectroscopic imaging. Am J Psychiatry 1996;153(12):1554–63.
97. Bertolino A, Saunders RC, Mattay VS, et al. Altered development of prefrontal neurons in rhesus monkeys with neonatal mesial temporo-limbic lesions: a proton magnetic resonance spectroscopic imaging study. Cereb Cortex 1997;7(8):740–8.
98. Lipska BK, Chrapusta SJ, Egan MF, et al. Neonatal excitotoxic ventral hippocampal damage alters dopamine response to mild repeated stress and to chronic haloperidol. Synapse 1995;20(2):125–30.
99. Lipska BK, Jaskiw GE, Chrapusta S, et al. Ibotenic acid lesion of the ventral hippocampus differentially affects dopamine and its metabolites in the nucleus accumbens and prefrontal cortex in the rat. Brain Res 1992;585(1–2):1–6.
100. Lipska BK, Jaskiw GE, Weinberger DR. Postpubertal emergence of hyperresponsiveness to stress and to amphetamine after neonatal excitotoxic hippocampal

damage: a potential animal model of schizophrenia. Neuropsychopharmacology 1993;9(1):67–75.

101. Lipska BK, Jaskiw GE, Weinberger DR. The effects of combined prefrontal cortical and hippocampal damage on dopamine-related behaviors in rats. Pharmacol Biochem Behav 1994;48(4):1053–7.
102. Lipska BK, Swerdlow NR, Geyer MA, et al. Neonatal excitotoxic hippocampal damage in rats causes post-pubertal changes in prepulse inhibition of startle and its disruption by apomorphine. Psychopharmacologia 1995;122(1):35–43.
103. Lipska BK, Weinberger DR. Genetic variation in vulnerability to the behavioral effects of neonatal hippocampal damage in rats. Proc Natl Acad Sci U S A 1995;92(19):8906–10.
104. Marsh L, Suddath RL, Higgins N, et al. Medial temporal lobe structures in schizophrenia: relationship of size to duration of illness. Schizophr Res 1994; 11(3):225–38.
105. Suddath RL, Christison GW, Torrey EF, et al. Anatomical abnormalities in the brains of monozygotic twins discordant for schizophrenia. N Engl J Med 1990;322(12):789–94.
106. Weinberger DR. Implications of normal brain development for the pathogenesis of schizophrenia. Arch Gen Psychiatry 1987;44(7):660–9.
107. Weinberger DR, Zigun JR, Bartley AJ, et al. Anatomical abnormalities in the brains of monozygotic twins discordant and concordant for schizophrenia. Clin Neuropharmacol 1992;15(Suppl 1 Pt A):122A–3A.
108. Martin A, Haxby JV, Lalonde FM, et al. Discrete cortical regions associated with knowledge of color and knowledge of action. Science 1995;270(5233): 102–5.
109. Schwarzlose RF, Baker CI, Kanwisher N. Separate face and body selectivity on the fusiform gyrus. J Neurosci 2005;25(47):11055–9.
110. Chao LL, Martin A, Haxby JV. Are face-responsive regions selective only for faces? Neuroreport 1999;10(14):2945–50.
111. Chao LL, Haxby JV, Martin A. Attribute-based neural substrates in temporal cortex for perceiving and knowing about objects. Nat Neurosci 1999;2(10):913–9.
112. Epstein R, Harris A, Stanley D, et al. The parahippocampal place area: recognition, navigation, or encoding? Neuron 1999;23(1):115–25.
113. Mahon BZ, Milleville SC, Negri GAL, et al. Action-related properties shape object representations in the ventral stream. Neuron 2007;55(3):507–20.
114. Morgan MA, Romanski LM, LeDoux JE. Extinction of emotional learning: contribution of medial prefrontal cortex. Neurosci Lett 1993;163(1):109–13.
115. Quirk GJ, Russo GK, Barron JL, et al. The role of ventromedial prefrontal cortex in the recovery of extinguished fear. J Neurosci 2000;20(16):6225–31.
116. Devinsky O, Morrell MJ, Vogt BA. Contributions of anterior cingulate cortex to behaviour. Brain 1995;118(Pt 1):279–306.
117. Bush G, Luu P, Posner MI. Cognitive and emotional influences in anterior cingulate cortex. Trends Cogn Sci 2000;4(6):215–22.
118. Vogt BA, Finch DM, Olson CR. Functional heterogeneity in cingulate cortex: the anterior executive and posterior evaluative regions. Cereb Cortex 1992;2(6): 435–43.
119. Whalen PJ, Bush G, McNally RJ, et al. The emotional counting Stroop paradigm: a functional magnetic resonance imaging probe of the anterior cingulate affective division. Biol Psychiatry 1998;44(12):1219–28.
120. Carter CS, Botvinick MM, Cohen JD. The contribution of the anterior cingulate cortex to executive processes in cognition. Rev Neurosci 1999;10(1):49–57.

121. Bush G, Whalen PJ, Rosen BR, et al. The counting Stroop: an interference task specialized for functional neuroimaging–validation study with functional MRI. Hum Brain Mapp 1998;6(4):270–82.
122. Bush G, Frazier JA, Rauch SL, et al. Anterior cingulate cortex dysfunction in attention-deficit/hyperactivity disorder revealed by fMRI and the counting Stroop. Biol Psychiatry 1999;45(12):1542–52.
123. Picard N, Strick PL. Motor areas of the medial wall: a review of their location and functional activation. Cereb Cortex 1996;6(3):342–53.
124. Rolls ET. The orbitofrontal cortex. Philos Trans R Soc Lond B Biol Sci 1996; 351(1346):1433–43 [discussion: 1443].
125. Damasio AR, Tranel D, Damasio H. Individuals with sociopathic behavior caused by frontal damage fail to respond autonomically to social stimuli. Behav Brain Res 1990;41(2):81–94.
126. Damasio A. A neural basis for sociopathy. Arch Gen Psychiatry 2000;57(2): 128–9.
127. de Zubicaray GI, Andrew C, Zelaya FO, et al. Motor response suppression and the prepotent tendency to respond: a parametric fMRI study. Neuropsychologia 2000;38(9):1280–91.
128. Horn NR, Dolan M, Elliott R, et al. Response inhibition and impulsivity: an fMRI study. Neuropsychologia 2003;41(14):1959–66.
129. Kawashima R, Satoh K, Itoh H, et al. Functional anatomy of GO/NO-GO discrimination and response selection–a PET study in man. Brain Res 1996;728(1): 79–89.
130. Liddle PF, Kiehl KA, Smith AM. Event-related fMRI study of response inhibition. Hum Brain Mapp 2001;12(2):100–9.
131. Watanabe J, Sugiura M, Sato K, et al. The human prefrontal and parietal association cortices are involved in NO-GO performances: an event-related fMRI study. Neuroimage 2002;17(3):1207–16.
132. Garavan H, Ross TJ, Murphy K, et al. Dissociable executive functions in the dynamic control of behavior: inhibition, error detection, and correction. Neuroimage 2002;17(4):1820–9.
133. Konishi S, Nakajima K, Uchida I, et al. Common inhibitory mechanism in human inferior prefrontal cortex revealed by event-related functional MRI. Brain 1999; 122(Pt 5):981–91.
134. Gruber SA, Rogowska J, Holcomb P, et al. Stroop performance in normal control subjects: an fMRI study. Neuroimage 2002;16(2):349–60.
135. Humberstone M, Sawle GV, Clare S, et al. Functional magnetic resonance imaging of single motor events reveals human presupplementary motor area. Ann Neurol 1997;42(4):632–7.
136. Rubia K, Russell T, Overmeyer S, et al. Mapping motor inhibition: conjunctive brain activations across different versions of go/no-go and stop tasks. Neuroimage 2001;13(2):250–61.
137. Stein DJ, Hollander E, Liebowitz MR. Neurobiology of impulsivity and the impulse control disorders. J Neuropsychiatry Clin Neurosci 1993;5(1):9–17.
138. Posner MI, Rothbart MK, Vizueta N, et al. An approach to the psychobiology of personality disorders. Dev Psychopathol 2003;15(4):1093–106.
139. Mostofsky SH, Schafer JGB, Abrams MT, et al. fMRI evidence that the neural basis of response inhibition is task-dependent. Brain Res Cogn Brain Res 2003;17(2):419–30.
140. Frith U, Frith CD. Development and neurophysiology of mentalizing. Philos Trans R Soc Lond B Biol Sci 2003;358(1431):459–73.

141. Fletcher PC, Happé F, Frith U, et al. Other minds in the brain: a functional imaging study of "theory of mind" in story comprehension. Cognition 1995; 57(2):109–28.
142. Gallagher HL, Happé F, Brunswick N, et al. Reading the mind in cartoons and stories: an fMRI study of 'theory of mind' in verbal and nonverbal tasks. Neuropsychologia 2000;38(1):11–21.
143. Vogeley K, Bussfeld P, Newen A, et al. Mind reading: neural mechanisms of theory of mind and self-perspective. Neuroimage 2001;14(1 Pt 1):170–81.
144. Brunet E, Sarfati Y, Hardy-Baylé MC, et al. A PET investigation of the attribution of intentions with a nonverbal task. Neuroimage 2000;11(2):157–66.
145. Goel V, Grafman J, Sadato N, et al. Modeling other minds. Neuroreport 1995; 6(13):1741–6.
146. Berthoz S, Armony JL, Blair RJR, et al. An fMRI study of intentional and unintentional (embarrassing) violations of social norms. Brain 2002;125(Pt 8):1696–708.
147. Castelli F, Happé F, Frith U, et al. Movement and mind: a functional imaging study of perception and interpretation of complex intentional movement patterns. Neuroimage 2000;12(3):314–25.
148. Schultz RT, Grelotti DJ, Klin A, et al. The role of the fusiform face area in social cognition: implications for the pathobiology of autism. Philos Trans R Soc Lond B Biol Sci 2003;358(1430):415–27.
149. Barnes CL, Pandya DN. Efferent cortical connections of multimodal cortex of the superior temporal sulcus in the rhesus monkey. J Comp Neurol 1992;318(2):222–44.
150. Allison T, Puce A, McCarthy G. Social perception from visual cues: role of the STS region. Trends Cogn Sci 2000;4(7):267–78.
151. Puce A, Perrett D. Electrophysiology and brain imaging of biological motion. Philos Trans R Soc Lond B Biol Sci 2003;358(1431):435–44.
152. Grezes J. Does perception of biological motion rely on specific brain regions? Neuroimage 2001;13(5):775–85.
153. Calvert GA, Campbell R, Brammer MJ. Evidence from functional magnetic resonance imaging of crossmodal binding in the human heteromodal cortex. Curr Biol 2000;10(11):649–57.
154. Campbell R, MacSweeney M, Surguladze S, et al. Cortical substrates for the perception of face actions: an fMRI study of the specificity of activation for seen speech and for meaningless lower-face acts (gurning). Brain Res Cogn Brain Res 2001;12(2):233–43.
155. McCabe K, Houser D, Ryan L, et al. A functional imaging study of cooperation in two-person reciprocal exchange. Proc Natl Acad Sci U S A 2001;98(20):11832–5.
156. Gallagher HL, Jack AI, Roepstorff A, et al. Imaging the intentional stance in a competitive game. Neuroimage 2002;16(3 Pt 1):814–21.
157. Williams LM, Brown KJ, Das P, et al. The dynamics of cortico-amygdala and autonomic activity over the experimental time course of fear perception. Brain Res Cogn Brain Res 2004;21(1):114–23.
158. Taylor SF, Phan KL, Decker LR, et al. Subjective rating of emotionally salient stimuli modulates neural activity. Neuroimage 2003;18(3):650–9.
159. Ochsner KN, Bunge SA, Gross JJ, et al. Rethinking feelings: an FMRI study of the cognitive regulation of emotion. J Cogn Neurosci 2002;14(8):1215–29.
160. Lane RD, Fink GR, Chau PM, et al. Neural activation during selective attention to subjective emotional responses. Neuroreport 1997;8(18):3969–72.
161. Gusnard DA, Akbudak E, Shulman GL, et al. Medial prefrontal cortex and self-referential mental activity: relation to a default mode of brain function. Proc Natl Acad Sci U S A 2001;98(7):4259–64.

162. Petrovic P, Ingvar M. Imaging cognitive modulation of pain processing. Pain 2002;95(1–2):1–5.
163. Frith CD, Frith U. Interacting minds–a biological basis. Science 1999;286(5445): 1692–5.
164. Etkin A, Pittenger C, Polan HJ, et al. Toward a neurobiology of psychotherapy: basic science and clinical applications. J Neuropsychiatry Clin Neurosci 2005;17(2):145–58.
165. Roffman JL, Marci CD, Glick DM, et al. Neuroimaging and the functional neuroanatomy of psychotherapy. Psychol Med 2005;35(10):1385–98.
166. Porto PR, Oliveira L, Mari J, et al. Does cognitive behavioral therapy change the brain? A systematic review of neuroimaging in anxiety disorders. J Neuropsychiatry Clin Neurosci 2009;21(2):114–25.
167. Beutel ME, Stark R, Pan H, et al. Changes of brain activation pre- post short-term psychodynamic inpatient psychotherapy: an fMRI study of panic disorder patients. Psychiatry Res 2010;184(2):96–104.
168. de Greck M, Scheidt L, Bölter AF, et al. Multimodal psychodynamic psychotherapy induces normalization of reward related activity in somatoform disorder. World J Biol Psychiatry 2011;12(4):296–308.
169. Gerber AJ, Kocsis JH, Milrod BL, et al. A quality-based review of randomized controlled trials of psychodynamic psychotherapy. Am J Psychiatry 2011; 168(1):19–28.
170. Lisiecka D, Meisenzahl E, Scheuerecker J, et al. Neural correlates of treatment outcome in major depression. Int J Neuropsychopharmacol 2011;14(4):521–34.
171. Ritchey M, Dolcos F, Eddington KM, et al. Neural correlates of emotional processing in depression: changes with cognitive behavioral therapy and predictors of treatment response. J Psychiatr Res 2011;45(5):577–87.
172. Forbes EE, Olino TM, Ryan ND, et al. Reward-related brain function as a predictor of treatment response in adolescents with major depressive disorder. Cogn Affect Behav Neurosci 2010;10(1):107–18.
173. Konarski JZ, Kennedy SH, Segal ZV, et al. Predictors of nonresponse to cognitive behavioural therapy or venlafaxine using glucose metabolism in major depressive disorder. J Psychiatry Neurosci 2009;34(3):175–80.
174. Siegle GJ, Carter CS, Thase ME. Use of FMRI to predict recovery from unipolar depression with cognitive behavior therapy. Am J Psychiatry 2006;163(4): 735–8.
175. Mayberg HS, Brannan SK, Mahurin RK, et al. Cingulate function in depression: a potential predictor of treatment response. Neuroreport 1997;8(4):1057–61.
176. Goldapple K, Segal Z, Garson C, et al. Modulation of cortical-limbic pathways in major depression: treatment-specific effects of cognitive behavior therapy. Arch Gen Psychiatry 2004;61(1):34–41.
177. Kumari V, Peters ER, Fannon D, et al. Dorsolateral prefrontal cortex activity predicts responsiveness to cognitive-behavioral therapy in schizophrenia. Biol Psychiatry 2009;66(6):594–602.
178. Koutsouleris N, Meisenzahl EM, Davatzikos C, et al. Use of neuroanatomical pattern classification to identify subjects in at-risk mental states of psychosis and predict disease transition. Arch Gen Psychiatry 2009;66(7):700–12.
179. Squire LR. Neuroscience. Rapid consolidation. Science 2007;316(5821):57–8.
180. Tse D, Langston RF, Kakeyama M, et al. Schemas and memory consolidation. Science 2007;316(5821):76–82.
181. Rumelhart D, Smolensky P, McClelland JL, et al. Schemata and sequential thought processes in PDP models. In: McClelland JL, Rumelhart DE, editors.

Parallel distributed processing: explorations in the microstructure of cognition. Volume 2: psychological and biological models. Cambridge (MA): MIT Press; 1986. p. 7–57.

182. van Kesteren MT, Fernández G, Norris DG, et al. Persistent schema-dependent hippocampal-neocortical connectivity during memory encoding and postencoding rest in humans. Proc Natl Acad Sci U S A 2010;107(16):7550–5.
183. Ding SL, Van Hoesen GW, Cassell MD, et al. Parcellation of human temporal polar cortex: a combined analysis of multiple cytoarchitectonic, chemoarchitectonic, and pathological markers. J Comp Neurol 2009;514(6):595–623.
184. Gotts SJ, Milleville SC, Bellgowan PS, et al. Broad and narrow conceptual tuning in the human frontal lobes. Cereb Cortex 2011;21(2):477–91.
185. Martin A, Weisberg J. Neural foundations for understanding social and mechanical concepts. Cogn Neuropsychol 2003;20(3–6):575–87.
186. Olson IR, Plotzker A, Ezzyat Y. The Enigmatic temporal pole: a review of findings on social and emotional processing. Brain 2007;130(Pt 7):1718–31.
187. Barsalou LW. Perceptual symbol systems. Behav Brain Sci 1999;22(4):577–609 [discussion: 610].
188. Niedenthal PM, Barsalou LW, Winkielman P, et al. Embodiment in attitudes, social perception, and emotion. Pers Soc Psychol Rev 2005;9(3):184–211.
189. Gallace A, Spence C. The cognitive and neural correlates of tactile memory. Psychol Bull 2009;135(3):380–406.
190. Mesulam MM. From sensation to cognition. Brain 1998;121(Pt 6):1013–52.
191. Andersen SM, Baum A. Transference in interpersonal relations: inferences and affect based on significant-other representations. J Pers 1994;62(4):459–97.
192. Andersen SM, Chen S. The relational self: an interpersonal social-cognitive theory. Psychol Rev 2002;109(4):619–45.
193. Gerber AJ, Peterson BS. Measuring transference phenomena with fMRI [abstract]. J Am Psychoanal Assoc 2006;54(4):1319–25.
194. McCleery JP, Ceponiene R, Burner KM, et al. Neural correlates of verbal and nonverbal semantic integration in children with autism spectrum disorders. J Child Psychol Psychiatry 2010;51(3):277–86.
195. Kamio Y, Toichi M. Memory illusion in high-functioning autism and Asperger's disorder. J Autism Dev Disord 2007;37(5):867–76.
196. Happé F, Briskman J, Frith U. Exploring the cognitive phenotype of autism: weak "central coherence" in parents and siblings of children with autism: I. Experimental tests. J Child Psychol Psychiat 2001;42(3):299–307.
197. Happe F, Booth RD. The power of the positive: revisiting weak coherence in autism spectrum disorders. Q J Psychol (Hove) 2008;61(1):50–63.
198. Mottron L, Burack JA, Iarocci G, et al. Locally oriented perception with intact global processing among adolescents with high-functioning autism: evidence from multiple paradigms. J Child Psychol Psychiatry 2003;44(6):904–13.
199. Fink GR, Marshall JC, Halligan PW, et al. Hemispheric specialization for global and local processing: the effect of stimulus category. Proc Biol Sci 1997; 264(1381):487–94.
200. Navon D. Forest before trees: the precedence of global features in visual perception. Cogn Psychol 1977;9:353–83.
201. Jolliffe T, Baron-Cohen S. Are people with autism and Asperger syndrome faster than normal on the embedded figures test? J Child Psychol Psychiatry 1997; 38(5):527–34.
202. Bolte S. Gestalt perception and local-global processing in high-functioning autism. J Autism Dev Disord 2007;37(8):1493–504.

203. Ring HA, Baron-Cohen S, Wheelwright S, et al. Cerebral correlates of preserved cognitive skills in autism: a functional MRI study of embedded figures task performance. Brain 1999;122(Pt 7):1305–15.
204. Granholm E, Cadenhead K, Shafer KM, et al. Lateralized perceptual organization deficits on the global-local task in schizotypal personality disorder. J Abnorm Psychol 2002;111(1):42–52.
205. Baxter LR Jr, Schwartz JM, Bergman KS, et al. Caudate glucose metabolic rate changes with both drug and behavior therapy for obsessive-compulsive disorder. Arch Gen Psychiatry 1992;49(9):681–9.
206. Bor J, Brunelin J, d'Amato T, et al. How can cognitive remediation therapy modulate brain activations in schizophrenia? An fMRI study. Psychiatry Res 2011; 192(3):160–6.
207. Brody AL, Saxena S, Stoessel P, et al. Regional brain metabolic changes in patients with major depression treated with either paroxetine or interpersonal therapy: preliminary findings. Arch Gen Psychiatry 2001;58(7):631–40.
208. de Lange FP, Koers A, Kalkman JS, et al. Increase in prefrontal cortical volume following cognitive behavioural therapy in patients with chronic fatigue syndrome. Brain 2008;131(Pt 8):2172–80.
209. Furmark T, Tillfors M, Marteinsdottir I, et al. Common changes in cerebral blood flow in patients with social phobia treated with citalopram or cognitive-behavioral therapy. Arch Gen Psychiatry 2002;59(5):425–33.
210. Goldin PR, Gross JJ. Effects of mindfulness-based stress reduction (MBSR) on emotion regulation in social anxiety disorder. Emotion 2010;10(1):83–91.
211. Goossens L, Sunaert S, Peeters R, et al. Amygdala hyperfunction in phobic fear normalizes after exposure. Biol Psychiatry 2007;62(10):1119–25.
212. Haut KM, Lim KO, MacDonald A 3rd. Prefrontal cortical changes following cognitive training in patients with chronic schizophrenia: effects of practice, generalization, and specificity. Neuropsychopharmacology 2010;35(9): 1850–9.
213. Hoekzema E, Carmona S, Tremols V, et al. Enhanced neural activity in frontal and cerebellar circuits after cognitive training in children with attention-deficit/ hyperactivity disorder. Hum Brain Mapp 2010;31(12):1942–50.
214. Huyser C, Veltman DJ, Wolters LH, et al. Functional magnetic resonance imaging during planning before and after cognitive-behavioral therapy in pediatric obsessive-compulsive disorder. J Am Acad Child Adolesc Psychiatry 2010; 49(12):1238–48, 1248.e1–5.
215. Kennedy SH, Konarski JZ, Segal ZV, et al. Differences in brain glucose metabolism between responders to CBT and venlafaxine in a 16-week randomized controlled trial. Am J Psychiatry 2007;164(5):778–88.
216. Kumari V, Fannon D, Peters ER, et al. Neural changes following cognitive behaviour therapy for psychosis: a longitudinal study. Brain 2011;134(Pt 8): 2396–407.
217. Lindauer RJ, Booij J, Habraken JB, et al. Effects of psychotherapy on regional cerebral blood flow during trauma imagery in patients with post-traumatic stress disorder: a randomized clinical trial. Psychol Med 2008;38(4):543–54.
218. Martin SD, Martin E, Rai SS, et al. Brain blood flow changes in depressed patients treated with interpersonal psychotherapy or venlafaxine hydrochloride: preliminary findings. Arch Gen Psychiatry 2001;58(7):641–8.
219. Nakatani E, Nakgawa A, Ohara Y, et al. Effects of behavior therapy on regional cerebral blood flow in obsessive-compulsive disorder. Psychiatry Res 2003; 124(2):113–20.

220. Prasko J, Horacek J, Zalesky R, et al. The change of regional brain metabolism (18FDG PET) in panic disorder during the treatment with cognitive behavioral therapy or antidepressants. Neuro Endocrinol Lett 2004;25(5):340–8.
221. Sakai Y, Kumano H, Nishikawa M, et al. Changes in cerebral glucose utilization in patients with panic disorder treated with cognitive-behavioral therapy. Neuroimage 2006;33(1):218–26.
222. Saxena S, Gorbis E, O'Neill J, et al. Rapid effects of brief intensive cognitive-behavioral therapy on brain glucose metabolism in obsessive-compulsive disorder. Mol Psychiatry 2009;14(2):197–205.
223. Schwartz JM, Stoessel PW, Baxter LR, et al. Systematic changes in cerebral glucose metabolic rate after successful behavior modification treatment of obsessive-compulsive disorder. Arch Gen Psychiatry 1996;53(2):109–13.
224. Vollstadt-Klein S, Loeber S, Kirsch M, et al. Effects of cue-exposure treatment on neural cue reactivity in alcohol dependence: a randomized trial. Biol Psychiatry 2011;69(11):1060–6.
225. Vocks S, Schulte D, Busch M, et al. Changes in neuronal correlates of body image processing by means of cognitive-behavioural body image therapy for eating disorders: a randomized controlled fMRI study. Psychol Med 2011; 41(8):1651–63.
226. Yamanishi T, Nakaaki S, Omori IM, et al. Changes after behavior therapy among responsive and nonresponsive patients with obsessive-compulsive disorder. Psychiatry Res 2009;172(3):242–50.
227. Drevets WC, Videen TO, Price JL, et al. A functional anatomical study of unipolar depression. J Neurosci 1992;12(9):3628–41.
228. Abercrombie HC, Schaefer SM, Larson CL, et al. Metabolic rate in the right amygdala predicts negative affect in depressed patients. Neuroreport 1998; 9(14):3301–7.
229. Gorman JM, Liebowitz MR, Fyer A, et al. A neuroanatomical hypothesis for panic disorder. Am J Psychiatry 1989;146(2):148–61.
230. Gorman JM, Kent JM, Sullivan GM, et al. Neuroanatomical hypothesis of panic disorder, revised. Am J Psychiatry 2000;157(4):493–505.
231. Baxter LR Jr, Schwartz JM, Phelps ME, et al. Reduction of prefrontal cortex glucose metabolism common to three types of depression. Arch Gen Psychiatry 1989;46(3):243–50.
232. Ring HA, Bench CJ, Trimble MR, et al. Depression in Parkinson's disease. A positron emission study. Br J Psychiatry 1994;165(3):333–9.
233. Biver F, Goldman S, Delvenne V, et al. Frontal and parietal metabolic disturbances in unipolar depression. Biol Psychiatry 1994;36(6):381–8.
234. de Asis JM, Stern E, Alexopolous GS, et al. Hippocampal and anterior cingulate activation deficits in patients with geriatric depression. Am J Psychiatry 2001; 158(8):1321–3.
235. Sheline YI, Sanghavi M, Mintun MA, et al. Depression duration but not age predicts hippocampal volume loss in medically healthy women with recurrent major depression. J Neurosci 1999;19(12):5034–43.
236. Woolley CS, McEwen BS. Estradiol mediates fluctuation in hippocampal synapse density during the estrous cycle in the adult rat. J Neurosci 1992;12(7):2549–54.
237. Buchsbaum MS, Joseph W, Siegel BV, et al. Effect of sertraline on regional metabolic rate in patients with affective disorder. Biol Psychiatry 1997;41(1):15–22.
238. Bench CJ, Friston KJ, Brown RG, et al. The anatomy of melancholia–focal abnormalities of cerebral blood flow in major depression. Psychol Med 1992;22(3): 607–15.

239. Elliott R, Rubinsztein JS, Sahakian BJ, et al. The neural basis of mood-congruent processing biases in depression. Arch Gen Psychiatry 2002;59(7):597–604.
240. Rajkowska G. Histopathology of the prefrontal cortex in major depression: what does it tell us about dysfunctional monoaminergic circuits? Prog Brain Res 2000; 126:397–412.
241. Mayberg HS. Limbic-cortical dysregulation: a proposed model of depression. J Neuropsychiatry Clin Neurosci 1997;9(3):471–81.
242. Drevets WC, Price JL, Simpson JR, et al. Subgenual prefrontal cortex abnormalities in mood disorders. Nature 1997;386(6627):824–7.
243. Hirayasu Y, Shenton ME, Salisbury DF, et al. Subgenual cingulate cortex volume in first-episode psychosis. Am J Psychiatry 1999;156(7):1091–3.
244. Ongur D, Drevets WC, Price JL. Glial reduction in the subgenual prefrontal cortex in mood disorders. Proc Natl Acad Sci U S A 1998;95(22):13290–5.
245. Kumari V, Mitterschiffthaler MT, Teasdale JD, et al. Neural abnormalities during cognitive generation of affect in treatment-resistant depression. Biol Psychiatry 2003;54(8):777–91.
246. Morys JM, Bobek-Billewicz B, Dziewiatkowskim J, et al. A magnetic resonance volumetric study of the temporal lobe structures in depression. Folia Morphol (Warsz) 2003;62(4):347–52.
247. Baxter LR Jr, Phelps ME, Mazziotta JC, et al. Cerebral metabolic rates for glucose in mood disorders. Studies with positron emission tomography and fluorodeoxyglucose F 18. Arch Gen Psychiatry 1985;42(5):441–7.

The Contemporary Psychodynamic Developmental Perspective

Norka T. Malberg, PsyD[a,*], Linda C. Mayes, MD[b]

KEYWORDS

- Mentalization • Attachment • Developmental psychoanalysis
- Developmental psychopathology

KEY POINTS

- There is a shift toward a 2-person psychology approach that informs the understanding of psychopathology from a developmental perspective.
- Advance in the scientific understanding of the intersubjective experience (namely from social neuroscience) has fostered a greater deal of interdisciplinary collaboration and dialogue between developmental psychoanalysis and other fields.
- Attachment theory provides the opportunity for empiric and clinical knowledge to meet and integrate into more cohesive and systemic intervention for children and families.

THE PSYCHODYNAMIC DEVELOPMENTAL PERSPECTIVE: PAST AND PRESENT

A developmental perspective has been part of psychoanalytic theory and clinical thinking since its inception. Freud's "Three essays on sexuality" (1905) outlined his theory of psychosexual phases, introduced the idea of a staged developmental ontogeny for libidinal change and orientation and set the scene for what was to be a continuous reworking and evolution of his ideas in this area. Clinical experience, and later close observation of children in the war nurseries, shaped the theories that Freud, Anna Freud, and their followers put forward. Early on, the theoretical formulations were also affected by prevailing concepts and then-current notions from fields such as the physical sciences and neurology.[1] However, Freud's 1895 project seeking a unitary conception of mind and brain was suspended prematurely as a result of the primitive state of neuroscience at the time. This early turning away from the influence of other disciplines and a heavy reliance on insights from clinical practice and clinical intuition guided the evolution of psychodynamic theory and its applications during most of the 20th century. This departure from integration with other disciplines also may have contributed to the prevalent perception of psychoanalysis as not adhering to a scientific method for advancement of the field and for not possessing a robust evidence base.

[a] Private Practice and Clinical Faculty, Yale Child Study Center, 147 Bishop Street, New Haven, CT 06525, USA; [b] Yale Child Study Center, 230 South Frontage Road, New Haven, CT 06519, USA
* Corresponding author.
E-mail address: norka.malberg@yale.edu

Child Adolesc Psychiatric Clin N Am 22 (2013) 33–49
http://dx.doi.org/10.1016/j.chc.2012.08.002 **childpsych.theclinics.com**

Abbreviations: Psychodynamic Developmental Perspective	
AAI	Adult Attachment Interview
CPP	Child-Parent Psychotherapy
MBT-A	Mentalization Based Therapy - Adolescents
MBTG-A	Mentalization Based Group Therapy for Adolescents
PIP	Parent Infant Project

Contemporary psychoanalytic writers in the developmental tradition have identified this turning away from the influence of other disciplines, and almost exclusive reliance on clinical observation and intuition, as a threat to the healthy evolution and survival of a psychodynamic approach to developmental psychopathology in the 21st century.[2] As a result, they emphasize the need for a radical reappraisal of psychoanalysis' epistemic framework in response to the current trends emerging from developmental psychopathology.

Developmental psychopathology focuses on the interplay between normality and pathology. Emphasizing a developmental framework for comprehending adaptation and maladaptation across the life course, developmental psychopathology pursues multiple levels of analysis and a multidomain approach to mapping development.[3–5] Many of the basic tenets guiding developmental psychopathology are present in the work of pioneers of the psychodynamic developmental tradition, such as Anna Freud. Anna Freud struggled with the complex metapsychological question: What moves development along, and is it inherently progressive and linear?[6] It could be argued that in essence, all of the psychoanalytic developmental theories are grounded in these basic tenets: understanding the interplay between normality and pathology; mapping multiple domains developing simultaneously; and taking a life course perspective.

The contemporary psychodynamic developmental perspective has set itself the challenging and ambitious agenda of becoming a more explicitly integrative, developmental psychopathological model of development from early infancy on through old age. By *integrative*, we mean several things:

1. Integration of earlier psychoanalytic theories with contemporary ideas
2. Integration of the many disciplines that study development: biology, neurology, cognitive and affective neuroscience, psychology, and education
3. Focusing not solely on an individual but also on the many systems that the individual functions within

Contemporary psychodynamic perspectives on development are also systemic, that is, understanding development as an interaction between endowment and environment (all social support systems surrounding the child). This theoretical shift departs from a classical view in which development is enshrined in stages and regression and psychosexual fixation are interpreted concretely, and moves toward a view of development as a consequence of the continuous interaction between the person (in terms of psychology and endowment) and the environment (in terms of the relationship between the person and social systems) To predict development under this transactional model, one must examine a system of interactional exchanges and continual restructuring of individual psychology based on these exchanges.[7]

Advances in the fields of cognitive and social neuroscience and genetics have informed this progression toward a more flexible, integrative, and systemic developmental psychodynamic approach. In this context, psychoanalytic theory, as pointed out by Fonagy and colleagues (2002),[8] provides an essential counterweight to advances in neuroscience and molecular genetics, preventing the oversimplification of the study of mental disorders and normative lifespan development.

In recent years, different psychoanalytic schools of thought have converged in the effort to formulate psychoanalysis as a relational theory. These approaches share, as a common thread, the belief that the human mind is interactive, that is, inherently social, rather than monadic, and that the psychoanalytic process should be understood as occurring between subjects rather than within the individual. From this perspective, mental life is seen through an intersubjective lens.[8,9] This shift over the last 25 years, in combination with the path-breaking work of researchers of infants[10,11] documenting intersubjectivity at the outset of human development, has contributed significantly to the emergence of a new brand of developmental psychoanalytic psychology: an interactional model, which, although retaining its focus on the investigation of mental processes as experienced and constructed from a subjective perspective, also lends itself to empiric inquiry through the integration of the explanatory lens of other disciplines including psychology, neuroscience, and genetics. A concrete example is the collaborative work of contemporary psychoanalysts, developmental psychologists, and cognitive neuroscientists in exploring the roots of adult borderline psychopathology through the lens of attachment theory and its measurable constructs.[8]

Here the authors highlight seminal contributions in contemporary developmental psychodynamic thinking and the treatment approaches these contributions foster. This new brand of developmental psychoanalysis seeks to produce empiric evidence that informs our understanding of the importance of the quality of the complex interactions whereby children and their environments shape each other. It also seeks to bring the empiric approach to the evaluation of treatments developed from the integration of clinical experience, basic research in psychology and neuroscience, and systemic analysis of the child's environment. Moving away from a monadic perspective to a relational and systemic view has facilitated development of psychotherapeutic interventions in outreach settings, such as schools and prisons.

CLINICAL APPLICATIONS EXEMPLIFYING THE CONTEMPORARY PSYCHODYNAMIC DEVELOPMENTAL PERSPECTIVE

An example of contemporary child psychoanalysis is the work of Jack Novick and Kerry Kelly Novick (2010)[12] in the United States. Their work, addressing the need for a more defined framework for working with parents, is remarkably relevant in the contemporary context in which an ecological approach to treatment has become indispensable (strengthening all primary social supports surrounding the child) The Novicks have recently coined the phrase *emotional muscle* (ego strength) to communicate to parents their pivotal role in their child's ego development. By doing so, they have embraced the challenging task of translating psychoanalytic thinking from a technical language into a language parents and teachers can understand. By helping these adults view the child through a developmental lens, they aim to effect significant shifts in the way the significant adults in a child's environment understand and respond to a child's emotional and behavioral struggles from a developmentally informed stance.

Another example is found in the work of the Parent Infant Project at the Anna Freud Center. This project illustrates the increased awareness of the need, in the era of increasing health care costs and evidence-based medicine, to tailor the theory and clinical practice of psychodynamic psychotherapy to the needs of specific populations (in this case, parents and their infants) or to use in specific environments to increase efficiency and effectiveness of treatment delivery (hostels, community settings, and prisons). This means that psychodynamic psychotherapy is offered to populations heretofore not always considered amendable to insight-oriented approaches (eg, families in prisons, single adolescent mothers) and in settings outside the contained and controlled consulting room (homeless shelters, prisons). Furthermore, their work reflects a departure from the monadic focus on internal conflicts so prominent in the work of 20th century child psychoanalysts, such as Anna Freud and Melanie Klein. There is a new emphasis on the integration of theory and technique to identify specific components of technique that are particularly effective with specific groups of children.

The work of the Parent Infant Project (2005) exemplifies a tendency in contemporary child analysis to develop interventions that can be manualized and replicated. This project, nested within the Anna Freud Center's developmental tradition, integrates the classical components of psychoanalytic intervention, such as the use of interpretation and verbalization of conflicting affects, with a relationally based approach to the emotional needs of parents and their infants informed by neuropsychology and developmental psychology.[13] The Parent Infant Project model, initially developed within the confines of the consulting room, has now been replicated in hostels and prisons[14] and represents a real example of the contemporary psychodynamic developmental perspective's emphasis on integration and of developmental psychoanalytic practice in the trenches. Furthermore, this new brand of psychodynamic psychotherapy, in the words of child psychoanalyst Anne Alvarez, is characterized by "the development of a meta-theory which is more relational, less reductionistic and mechanistic and more able to accommodate novelty, growth, change and the awareness of mind."[15,16]

CONTEMPORARY PSYCHODYNAMIC DEVELOPMENTAL THEORY INTEGRATES THE TRADITIONAL PSYCHOANALYTIC PERSPECTIVE WITH NEW RESEARCH

The developmental psychodynamic perspective has been influenced and transformed in the last 2 decades by developments in neuroscience,[17] an increasing awareness of the clinical applications of attachment theory,[8] and the emergence of clinical research focusing on parent-infant interactions.[18] These new developments enrich the traditional psychoanalytic developmental perspectives from the work of child psychoanalytic thinkers, such as Winnicott, Mahler, Anna Freud, and Melanie Klein. Their conceptualizations of the internal world of the child in the context of object relations continue to provide a strong theoretical framework and inform the development of new ways of organizing and integrating insights from both the clinic and research studies.

For instance, the contemporary concept of mentalization as elaborated by Bateman and Fonagy[19] integrates components of Winnicott's understanding of the importance of the quality of the first relationship with the evidence provided by contemporary research from the fields of attachment and neuropsychology. In the same way, Melanie Klein's clinical insights into the role of parental projections onto the infant inform the explanatory model of Bateman and Fonagy[19] of the dyadic process from which the borderline personality structure emerges.

Margaret Mahler's work (1975)[20] regarding the process of separation and individuation in the context of the parent-child dyadic relationship provides a frame to observe what contemporary writers such as Stern[11] call the relational dance between mother and young child. Finally, when considered in the context of environmental influences, Anna Freud's understanding of the fluid nature of development, as exemplified by her concept of the developmental line, sets the stage for contemporary transactional models of development.[7] Thus, contemporary psychodynamic thinking has been able to incorporate concepts that have emerged from detailed clinical observation and integrate and validate them within a more comprehensive and flexible theoretical working model.

Contemporary psychoanalytic developmental theory also emerges from an object relations tradition in which psychological development is viewed as occurring in an interpersonal matrix.[21] Coming from this interpersonal angle, contemporary developmentalists have tapped into the rich vein of research on attachment. The work of attachment researchers such as Mary Main and colleagues [22–24] has provided empiric support to Bowlby and Ainsworth's[25,26] original observations regarding the importance of the quality of the primary caregiver relationship. Furthermore, it has enabled contemporary psychodynamic thinkers to explore innovative ways of integrating empiric findings into the design and implementation of clinical interventions.

An example of such integration is the work of Alicia Lieberman,[27] who developed Child-Parent Psychotherapy, informed by the findings of attachment research and the work of child psychoanalyst Selma Fraiberg,[28–30] on the intergenerational transmission of trauma. Lieberman's work has been applied to the needs of specific clinical populations such as depressed mothers of toddlers.[31] The interventions described by Toth and colleagues[31] focus on preventing the adverse longitudinal impact of maternal depression on young children. This aim is achieved by focusing on the activation of the mother's reflective functioning found through extensive research to be a strong mediator of attachment outcome in children.[32] Reflective functioning refers to the mother's capacity to make sense of her young child's internal experience by using her understanding of the child's mental states (intentions, feelings, thoughts, desires, and beliefs). Healthy capacity for reflective function lets the mother effectively anticipate, perceive, and respond to the mental states driving the child's behavior. A mother's reflective function allows her to anticipate, be curious about, and understand (or guess) with more accuracy what the child wants and needs. Another way of thinking about reflective function is that it allows the mother to understand which mental states belong to her and which belong to her child. If all has gone well in her own development, a mother/parent has the capacity to think of the young child as separate, with his or her own emotional needs and states of mind that are nonetheless highly responsive to the parent's emotional states.

Bowlby, a psychoanalyst himself, felt that actual events such as loss and separation and the internal experience of loss/separation, affected the development of the child and the later functioning of the adult.[33] He emphasized the importance of understanding infant-mother attachment as based on a primary and autonomous instinctual system instead of a derivative of the drives. Because it emerged through observations of real-life separations and losses in childhood, attachment theory reflects the emphasis on an integrative view of human development that brings together internal and external experience, relationships among children and adults, and a broader systemic view of a child's developmental environment.

Contemporary clinical researchers, working through the attachment lens and working within the developmental psychodynamic tradition, such as Steele and Steele,[34] and Strathearn and colleagues[35] have built on the efforts of Mary Ainsworth (1969)[36] who operationalized the study of the effect the quality of maternal care has on the development of the child's patterns of attachment. Ainsworth's work on patterns of attachment in the Strange Situation and Mary Main's work on the Adult Attachment Interview were pivotal in translating Bowlby's theoretical contributions into operationalized and empiric language and facilitated a bridge between contemporary attachment research and developmental psychoanalysis.

Mary Main's research using the Adult Attachment Interview first suggested that a child's metacognitive capacity, that is, the ability to reflect on one's experiences, serves as a significant psychological protective factor. However, many of the follow-up studies[37,38] focused on the importance of a mother's capacity to regulate and organize thoughts and feelings about her own childhood history of receiving care and this capacity's link to her ability to regulate, organize, and respond sensitively to her child's attachment needs (comfort, safety, and closeness). This was a significant shift toward an emphasis on the impact of the quality of the relationship on the child's emotional and social development and on defining a developmental environment.

THE MENTALIZATION CONSTRUCT: AN EXAMPLE OF THE INTEGRATION OF THEORIES AND RESEARCH IN THE EVOLUTION FROM THE TRADITIONAL TO THE CONTEMPORARY PSYCHODYNAMIC DEVELOPMENTAL PERSPECTIVE

Following on the work of the attachment researchers, Fonagy and colleagues,[39] in an attempt to integrate psychoanalytic ideas with emerging findings from the fields of social cognition, neuroscience, and attachment research defined the construct of mentalization, namely, the capacity to understand the behaviors of self and others in terms of underlying mental states and intentions. The mentalization-based approach to psychotherapy has emerged as an integrative model that provides the clinician with a new lens through which to observe clinical phenomena and construct case formulations.

Mentalization, developed as an empirically testable construct, is measured as reflective functioning, an overt manifestation in narrative of an individual's mentalizing capacity.[32] A primary caregiver who is able to hold on to complex mental states is able to hold her child's internal affective experience in mind, thereby facilitating her understanding of her child's behavior with respect to his or her own feelings and intentions. The caregiver functioning from this reflective stance imparts meaning to the child's affective experiences in a way that promotes regulation. In this way, a caregiver fosters emotional security in her child. Mentalization capacity in the caregiver is vital to maintain and facilitate a range of progressive developmental processes in the child. Consequently, the absence of this experience of parental reflective functioning is seen as underlying the development of various forms of psychopathology.[8] By operationalizing reflective functioning as a measure of mentalizing capacity and studying the impact of parental reflective function on a child's development, researchers have shown the importance of the caregiver's mentalizing capacity in the developmental outcome of the child. This has shifted the attention of child psychoanalysts and psychodynamic therapists toward working with parents and the importance of exploring the personal meaning of parenting and how it influences reflective capacities.

The emerging field of cognitive neuroscience provides another source of support for the role of mentalization as development progresses in the context of relationships. Specifically, the neurologically based research taken up by attachment theorists[8,40,41] articulated the role of attunement in early relationships in the development of affect regulation and the capacity to engage in relationships. Strong evidence now shows the negative impact of neglectful or abusive early relationships on development and an association with a diverse range of adverse neurodevelopmental outcomes, including long-term cognitive and academic delays[42] and on the overall development of a child's brain architecture.[43]

THE MENTALIZATION-BASED INTERVENTION

> *Psychoanalysis is the only psychological treatment which sets itself the ambitious goal of restructuring the components of the individual's adaptation, and aims to address all aspects of the patient's personality. Perhaps because of the scope of its ambitions, attempts at operationalizing the process and outcome of child analysis are at very early stages of development. (By operationalizing, we mean the explicit specification of aspects of the treatment, or of methods of recording information.)*[44]

Faced with the reality of a need for more evidence to support the efficacy of clinical treatments coupled with demands for shorter yet effective treatments, the mentalization-based approach to psychodynamic psychotherapy seeks to integrate principles from classical psychodynamic theory and technique, such as Anna Freud's understanding of the developmental nature of psychological defenses, with the contemporary psychodynamic developmental perspective grounded in research and clinical observation. Mentalization-based treatment reflects a trend toward achieving a stronger link between research and clinical practice and an integration of systemic understanding of child psychopathology into psychodynamic thinking.

Over the course of the 20th century, no clear definitions emerged to distinguish psychoanalysis from psychodynamic psychotherapy. The easiest distinction made between these 2 modalities had to do with the frequency of sessions (a psychoanalytic case had a minimum of 4 sessions weekly), whereas a psychodynamic psychotherapy intervention tended to range from once per week to twice per week. In addition, although the overall aims of both modalities were guided by the same overarching theoretical principles, the treatment goals themselves tended to be more ambitious for the psychoanalysis of a child, namely, a more focused effort on structural changes in the psyche. Technique also differed in that the emergence of the transference in the consulting room was explored more deeply in psychoanalysis. Psychodynamic psychotherapy tended to be somewhat more focused on how specific aspects of the child's functioning obstructed or facilitated progressive development and adaptation to the challenges in the child's environment. With these distinctions between the 2 common modalities used with children, there are continued efforts to define and operationalize who can benefit from which modality and what the components are that define efficacious treatments.

As an initial response to this need, Fonagy and Target[44] carried out a retrospective review of 763 cases of children and adolescents treated at the Anna Freud Center with the aim of exploring the effectiveness of child psychodynamic treatment, but most importantly to determine which children seemed to benefit most from a most intensive psychoanalytic approach. Before this retrospective review, only a handful of studies had attempted to explore the effectiveness of insight-oriented treatments for children. Heinicke and Ramsey-Klee[45] had evaluated psychoanalytic treatment for latency children referred for learning disturbances and academic deficiencies. The frequency of treatment was either 1 or 4 sessions per week or a period at each frequency. The results of that study showed that both intensities of treatment led to gains in self-esteem, adaptation, and the capacity for relationships, but the gains were significantly greater and better maintained for the more intensive treatment. A second study by Moran and colleagues[46] examined the efficacy of child psychoanalytic interventions with children with brittle diabetes. A group of 11 patients treated in 3- to 4-times weekly psychoanalytic psychotherapy alongside medical management were compared with patients receiving the usual psychological assessment and medical management without any psychotherapy. The group treated with psychoanalytic psychotherapy showed significant improvement in blood glucose control: a strong indicator of the value of the intensive psychotherapy intervention. The psychotherapy had focused on the personal meaning of the illness and its impact on personality functioning and development. Central to the work was the development of a reliable and predictable intensive psychotherapeutic relationship.

The results of the retrospective study by Fonagy and Target[44] suggested that children with anxiety disorders (with or without comorbidity) showed greater improvement than those with other conditions and greater improvements than would be expected based on studies of untreated outcome.[47] More than 85% of 299 children with anxiety and depressive disorders no longer suffered any diagnosable emotional disorder after an average of 2 years of treatment. The study concluded that children with severe or pervasive symptoms, such as overanxious disorder, or comorbid disorders benefited from an intensive psychotherapy approach, whereas focused anxiety symptoms, such as phobias or obsessive-compulsive disorder, improved more or less equally with once- or twice-weekly sessions.

These studies suggested that the psychodynamic approach to working with children and adolescents is efficacious and effective. At the same time, these studies also underscored the need for operationalization and specificity of technique. In response to this, during the last 2 decades, psychodynamic treatment modalities have begun to integrate the clinical experience of the 20th century with an operationalized and, usually, manualized foundation. Mentalization-based treatment is an example of a treatment modality that includes both integrative and evidenced-based developmental psychodynamic framework.

Mentalization-based treatment is based on the mentalization construct, that is, understanding one's own and another's mental states as measured by reflective functioning, as a foundation for a psychodynamic therapy that can be further operationalized and thus more readily manualized. Most of the interventions included in mentalization-based therapy seek to enhance the child's capacity to mentalize, but, most importantly, they also seek to activate the reflective functioning capacities of the systems (family, school, hospital) supporting the child in his efforts to achieve progressive development. In other words, the mentalization-based approach with children and adolescents seeks to[48–50]:

- Enhance reflective processes (perspective taking, curiosity, and flexibility)
- Strengthen impulse control (affect regulation)
- Increase awareness of others as separate and intentional beings (inquisitive stance)
- Develop the capacity to play (playfulness and joyful moments)
- Work in parallel with, or in the context of, the systems supporting the child to activate reflective functioning (mentalizing the system)

By taking into consideration the child's attachment history and his past and current psychological and social functioning, this intervention, developed under a relational developmental approach, seeks to restore developmental progress and strengthen the child's capacity to function more effectively in relationships. This contemporary psychodynamic approach seeks to accomplish this goal by taking a more focused relational and ecological approach.

CLINICAL EXAMPLE: REFLECTIONS ON CONTEMPORARY PSYCHODYNAMIC TECHNIQUE IN THE OUTREACH CONTEXT

As early as 1966, Anna Freud, in her article, "Interactions between Nursery School and Child Guidance Clinic," highlighted the importance of establishing a dialogue between educators and child mental health providers. She spoke of the benefits of integrating the insights from clinical practice with those coming from education regarding children's learning and developmental processes in the context of schools. In the same fashion, she spoke of the importance of establishing further interdisciplinary dialogue with doctors, nurses, lawyers, and social workers.[51]

Contemporary developmental psychoanalysis has continued to develop interventions based on Anna Freud's goal of integrating knowledge from other fields to inform our practice. For example, recent findings[52] linking the impact of early relationships to development in the brain provides strong support for one of the basic tenets of the developmental psychodynamic school of thought, that of the importance of the child psychotherapist as a new developmental object with whom the child can relate in a different way. However, this research also sheds light on the importance of working with parents, teachers, and other people in the child's social support system to strengthen those relationships in a way that promotes the feeling of well being and growth in the child.

The following clinical example is an illustration of this cross-fertilization with other fields and the emergence of specific constructs from attachment theory, which inform our practice, enhancing our capacity to be effective in outreach contexts. This example comes from an early intervention project in the United Kingdom developed under the aegis of the Anna Freud Center and developed by child psychotherapists from the developmental psychodynamic tradition. The project aimed to promote the activation of reflective functioning in parents and teachers by inviting them to reflect on their own experiences and how they influence their understanding and responses to young children's challenging behaviors. The main goal of the Primary School Prevention Project is to prevent early exclusion from school. Early exclusion usually results from the educational system's incapacity to contain and manage a young child's behaviors and emotional difficulties. At the time of referral, the child is observed in the context of school and a series of diagnostic meetings take place with teachers, caregivers, and the child. The relationship between the child, his teacher, and his parents is observed through joint sessions. This evaluation informs the choice of treatment modality. The project offers short-term mentalization-based work with the child, parent-child sessions, joint meetings with teachers and parents, and individual parent meetings depending on the diagnostic formulation resulting from the initial meetings.

JOEY

Joey was referred by his kindergarten teacher. He was a sweet-looking 5 year old, who had recently become unmanageable in his classroom setting. He had begun to hit others and spit at teachers when disciplined, he refused to sit in circle time, and constantly defied the teacher's authority. His mother, a single 22-year-old woman from Sudan, felt at a loss for how to help her son. At home, Joey was well behaved, helpful, and very mindful of other people's feelings according to his mother. She described having stomach aches every morning worrying about Joey's behavior at school and being at work and becoming anxious every time her cell phone rang, fearing it was the school asking her to pick up her child. She was concerned about losing her job as a result, and spoke of her lack of social supports. Ms. Taylor, Joey's teacher, was a well-intentioned young teacher in her second year of practice who had become increasingly concerned about Joey's frequent school absences. Before beginning work with Joey, the therapist met with both Joey's mother and Ms. Taylor to explore their understanding of Joey's difficulties. In addition, the therapist observed Joey's behavior in his classroom and in the playground. The Child Behavior Checklist and the Strengths and Difficulties inventory were also given to mother and teacher to monitor their perception and understanding of the child's difficulties. The therapist met twice with Joey and once with Joey and his mother to assess his ego functioning and developmental progress in general. Most importantly, the therapist arranged individual meetings with Joey to try to shed light onto his own understanding of his difficulties and how they influence the way he thought of himself in the context of relationships (eg, bad boy, unlovable?).

Joey related well to the therapist, he appeared contained and able to play and experience moments of shared joy with the therapist and his mother. However, on the playground, he struggled to read his peers' cues and seemed to be waiting "for the other shoe to drop" as described by Ms. Taylor. Similarly, in the context of the classroom, Joey seemed lost. He misread Ms. Taylor's feedback as punishing and persecutory, and, in response, he would retaliate by trying to assert his power physically.

The psychotherapist arranged weekly mother-child sessions in parallel with meetings with Joey's mother and Ms. Taylor. In addition, the therapist met individually with Joey every other week. As the work progressed, it became clear that Joey and his mother were socially isolated, and this had contributed to Joey's hunger for attention and exclusivity in all his relationships. Ms. Taylor began to communicate more with Joey's mother and include her as a volunteer in class during her day off from work. In addition, a plan to contain him so as not to call his mother so frequently was put in place, and Joey became part of a playgroup after school for young children with social skills difficulties. Joey flourished, and his mother became a very involved member of the school community. Ms. Taylor also began to help Joey's peers to see the "other Joey" by giving him leadership roles in the classroom. This represented a significant shift in her management of the child as she began to be able to reflect on the meaning of his behaviors instead of reacting to them, often in a punitive and, what she perceived as ineffective, fashion. During her consultations with the therapist, Ms. Taylor was able to explore her own emotional responses to Joey and reflect on how they influenced her understanding of the child and his behavior.

By providing a supportive reflective (mentalizing) environment for both Ms. Taylor and Joey's mother, the therapist was able to understand the emotional needs behind Joey's behaviors. His challenging behavior was a communication to the world regarding his mother's loneliness and anxiety and his sense of feeling burdened by it. On the other hand, by providing a secure base for his mother to explore her own past experiences and think about the impact of her struggles on her child, the therapist was able to give Joey's mother an emerging sense of agency (a voice) and activated her capacity to differentiate her own emotional needs from those of her child. As a result, Joey's mother was able to become a more confident and predictable parent and help her son feel safe and contained.

APPLICATION OF CONTEMPORARY DEVELOPMENTAL PSYCHODYNAMIC THEORY AND TECHNIQUE WITHIN THE CONTEXT OF MULTIMODAL TREATMENT PLANS

Joey's case is a good example of how contemporary research from attachment has integrated itself into a strong preexisting clinical psychodynamic developmental tradition. It provides the strength of a clear and evidence-based conceptual framework, one that considers the intrapersonal and interpersonal origins of challenging behavior and psychopathology and is guided by a fluid and flexible model of development. By assuming a systemic approach to clinical formulation and treatment planning, the clinician in this case was able to encourage the process of mentalizing the needs of the child in the family and the school system in the process encouraging a reflective and holding environment for the child and his difficulties.

Many of the components highlighted through the elaboration of Joey's case are present in additional models presented in the next sections. The following examples represent only a small sample of a larger shift in the application of psychodynamic developmental principles to the current needs of clinical populations and the social systems supporting them. There is an increasing acknowledgment of the need for interventions that are integrative, systemic, and, most importantly, replicable and accessible. Furthermore, these examples represent a shift from a focus on developing interventions based on work in the consulting room to the development of replicable applications developed based on the needs of specific systems (eg, hospitals and schools) and specific populations (eg, substance abusing mothers).

CLINICAL INTERVENTION EXAMPLE: THE MOTHERS AND TODDLERS PROGRAM

The Mothers and Toddlers Program[53] is an attachment-based parenting intervention for substance abusing mothers. The program offers a 20-week individual therapy intervention that aims to help substance-using mothers develop more balanced representations of their children and improve their capacity for reflective functioning. It seeks to intervene individually with mothers to improve their capacity to respond sensitively to their young children's cues, to respond to and soothe their children when distressed, and to foster the progressive social and emotional development of their children. All of these aims address characteristics of reflective functioning. The therapists focus on the mother's own expectations for her role as a parent and her own needs as she tries to understand both what it means to be a parent and what her infant/child needs. Before treatment, mothers' attachment patterns as well as the quality of their attributions regarding their children's behaviors are assessed. Clinicians also obtain a baseline measure of children's behavioral profiles. The intervention seeks to identify and address intergenerational patterns of insecure attachment behavior reflective of the parent's own troubled, neglectful, or abusive childhood. By tackling intergenerational transmission of representations, this intervention offers the opportunity for a new developmental experience to the parent, one that allows her to consider new ways of responding and interacting with her child and responding to her own feelings as a parent. As shown by the preliminary findings of this project, not only did mothers display improvement in their representational balance and reflective functioning capacities, but their children also showed significant improvements in their behavior and their overall socioemotional development.[53]

PEACEFUL SCHOOL PROJECT

"Connected, reflective people make safe non coercive communities"[54]

The Peaceful School Project is a good example of contemporary psychodynamic interventions serving the needs of children in their communities from a developmental psychodynamic perspective with a powerful systemic lens. Designed to address bullying, its major guiding psychological construct is mentalization. The project focuses on the importance of identifying unconscious power dynamics in the school system and the impact they have on the development of coercive social forces that reduce an individual's capacity to think in mental states. As a result, behavioral manifestations (aggressive actions) become the primary way of responding to a collective lack of felt agency within a nonmentalizing culture. This project works with teachers and other school personnel as well as with parents and their children and seeks to activate the capacity to identify what is behind the bullying behavior and shift the response of the home and school environment to the child toward a more mentalizing stance. In this way, the project accomplishes an increase sense of agency on all participants and fosters an ethos of "thinking about feeling and thinking about thinking" when confronted with nonthinking, aggressive behaviors.

Based on empiric evidence from the attachment field, Twemlow and colleagues[55] put forward the hypothesis that an integrative approach to intervention can have broad application to the understanding of social problems, such as violence and neglect of young children (eg, by attempting to mentalize the system through active and explicit identification of bullying patterns in the school system using the "helpful bystander" concept). The helpful bystander has the power to play a key role in preventing or stopping bullying directly by discouraging the bully, defending the victim, or redirecting the situation away from bullying. This project was able to highlight the impact of feeling recognized (seen and heard) on the child's capacity for self-regulation. As described by the authors: "feeling recognized as an individual creates an analogue of the secure base experience and permits the activation of associated mental models with confidence to experience distress knowing that it will not overwhelm or permanently dys-regulate one's one capacity to function."[55]

The project also tackles the question of how to collaborate and work with the supporting systems around the child, that is, parents and teachers. The Peaceful Schools Program offers long-term psychodynamic psychotherapy to both children and families and works actively with schools and teachers in identifying the patterns of behavior in staff and attitudes in the system that facilitate the emergence of bullying within the system. By choosing a clearly central construct, such as the concept of mentalization, a capacity central to all psychotherapeutic and human endeavors, the intervention provides clear goals and treatment planning around a main goal, that of activating the reflective capacities of the system and the child through a parallel relational process respectful of the developmental and psychosocial needs of all involved in the process. Furthermore, by creating a common and accessible language for everyone in the system, interdisciplinary collaboration is possible and effective.

CLINICAL APPLICATION WITH ADOLESCENTS AND THOSE SUPPORTING THEM

Working clinically with adolescents represents a challenge to the clinician, as many primitive states of minds, loaded with anxiety, are awakened in the clinician as well as in the supporting systems (eg, school staff, parents, pediatricians). Recently, a series of outcome studies have been developed to examine interventions with adolescents informed by both classical and contemporary developmental psychodynamic theory and technique. The authors briefly review the work with 2 challenging subsets of this population: self-harming and chronically ill adolescents.

An Intervention with Self-harming Adolescents

The work of Trudie Rossouw in the United Kingdom with self-harming adolescents from a mentalization-based approach has produced valuable clinical insights regarding the importance of integration of modalities when working with self-harming adolescents. One of the landmarks of her intervention is the exploration of what Fonagy has termed the alien self. The alien self is an internal representation that emerges in the context of a relational exchange filled with parental negative projections and little experience of a primary object attempting to have one's mind in their mind.[56] Like many other mentalization-based interventions, Rossouw's work[50] seeks to help the young person and his family improve his or her awareness of his or her own mental states and the mental states of others. The intervention integrates explicit and implicit techniques for encouraging the reflective capacities of the young person and the family. Family interventions consist of focused and experiential approaches to psychoeducation, insight, and modeling of a reflective and inquisitive stance in the psychotherapist. By working in the "here and now" with the young person and the family, the intervention seeks to provide a new relational experience for the young person and the family. Within this new relational experience, internal representations can be revisited, hopefully resulting in more coherent narratives of the self in the context of relationships and, most importantly, increasing a sense of agency. With this should come an improved capacity for mentalized affectivity, the ability to think while experiencing strong, activating feelings. Preliminary results show support of the initial clinical hypothesis with significant reduction of young people's self-harming behaviors and improvement of parent's reflective capacities.[48,50]

Working with Chronically Ill Adolescents

Like Rossouw, Norka Malberg's group works[48,50] with chronically ill adolescents, specifically young people experiencing end-stage renal disease who exhibit difficulties adhering to critical but onerous medical regimes. The mentalization-based group therapy for adolescents approach focuses on activating the capacity for reflective functioning in chronically ill adolescent patients by using a group modality. This 12-week intervention seeks to create a secure base, a relational laboratory, from which to explore the impact of chronic illness on the internal representations of the young patient. The intervention seeks to scaffold the process of activating reflective functioning while respecting the defensive structures needed to endure the stress and trauma provoked by the ongoing exposure to chronic illness. The intervention incorporates technical aspects of more classical psychodynamic interventions, such as explicit exploration of defensive strategies and open identification and verbalization of affects. However, the mentalization construct, and the language developed around it, provides a useful conduit for collaboration and parallel processes with parents and health professionals supporting the young person. Parenting groups and discussion groups with nurses in which participants are invited to mentalize around issues of medical adherence in the young patients are run parallel to the group work with the adolescents. Results of an initial pilot study showed significant improvement in biologic measures of medical adherence as well as reports of improved quality of interactions in the medical unit between parents, nurses, and patients.[57] These findings highlight the need for interventions that introduced a clearer developmental understanding of the emotional needs of chronically ill adolescents but also explore, in a structured and safe setting, the multiple meanings present in the relational exchanges surrounding the patient.

These projects, the Mothers and Toddlers Program, Peaceful Schools, mentalization-based therapy approach for self-harming adolescents, and a group therapy program for chronically ill adolescents, are examples of integration of theory and research from multiple disciplines and efforts to operationalize theoretical and technical constructs. Operationalization facilitates replication and promotion of interventions with an increasingly firm evidence base. These projects are the product of contemporary developmental psychodynamic thought.

SUMMARY

Here are reviewed the changes in psychodynamic approaches to child development over the last 8 decades since Anna Freud and others began applying psychoanalytic understanding to working therapeutically with children. Although Anna Freud and her colleagues initially were forced to work in real world settings as they helped children during the London blitz, much of the earliest psychodynamically oriented work with children occurred in the consulting room and playroom with careful attention to the meaning of the child's play and his or her emerging inner world. As psychodynamic developmental theory has evolved and taken on a developmental psychopathology perspective that acknowledges the constant interplay between biology/endowment and experience/environment, child psychoanalysts and developmentally oriented clinicians have once again returned to real world settings, including schools and hospitals, drug-treatment facilities, prisons, and community centers. Additionally, with the incorporation of attachment theory and mentalization perspectives has come a greater emphasis on a systematic perspective and on studying the impact of psychodynamically oriented treatments with children and families, operationalizing treatment approaches, and developing a robust evidence base. Data are accumulating regarding the implementation and impact of mentalization-based treatments. Child psychoanalysts and psychodynamically oriented clinicians are using a range of techniques borrowed from different treatment approaches and models of effectiveness. These new models, or approaches, to psychodynamic treatment with children and families or in community settings also necessarily require new approaches to training child mental health clinicians. Additionally, the contemporary psychodynamic developmental perspective offers better opportunities for collaborations across clinical disciplines, including developmental psychology and neuroscience.

REFERENCES

1. Sandler J, Holder A, Dare C, et al. Freud's models of the mind. London: Karnac Books; 1997.
2. Fonagy P, Target M. The place of psychodynamic theory in developmental psychopathology. Dev Psychopathol 2000;12:407–25.
3. Cichetti D. Development and psychopathology. In: Cohen DJ, Cichetti D, editors. Developmental psychopathology. New York: Wiley; 2004. p. 701–49.
4. Dubowitz H. Neglected children: research, practice & policy. Thousand Oaks, CA: Sage; 1999.
5. Fonagy P, Moran GS. Studies on the efficacy of child psychoanalysis. J Consult Clin Psychol 1990;58:684–95.
6. Mayes LC, Cohen DJ. Anna Freud and developmental psychoanalytic psychology. Psychoanal Study Child 1996;51:117–41.
7. Sameroff A. The transactional model of development: how children and context shape each other. Washington, DC: American Psychological Association; 2009.
8. Fonagy P, Gergely G, Jurist E, et al. Affect regulation, mentalization and the development of the self. New York: Other Press; 2002.
9. Benjamin J. An outline of intersubjectivity: the development of recognition. Psychoanal Psychol 1990;7:33–46.
10. Beebe B, Lachmann F. Mother-Infant mutual influence and precursors of psychic structure. In: Golberg A, editor. Frontiers in self psychology, progress in self-pathology, vol. 3. Hillsdale (NJ): Analytic Press; 1988. p. 3–25.
11. Stern D. The interpersonal world of the infant. London: Karnac Books; 1998.
12. Novick J, Kelly Novick K. Emotional muscle: strong parents, strong children. Ann Arbor, MI: Xlibris; 2010.
13. Trevarthen C, Aitken KJ. Infant intersubjectivity: Research, theory and clinical applications. J Child Psychol Psychiatry 2001;42:3–48.
14. Barandon T. Relational trauma in infancy: psychoanalytic, attachment and neuropsychological contributions to parent-infant psychotherapy. London, UK: Routledge; 2010.

15. Alvarez A. Live company: psychoanalytic psychotherapy with autistic, borderline, deprived and abused children. London, UK: Routledge; 1999.
16. Barandon T, Broughton C, Gibbs I, et al. The practice of psychoanalytic parent-infant psychotherapy: claiming the baby. London, UK: Routledge; 2005.
17. Schore AN. Affect regulation and the origin of the self: the neurobiology of emotional development. Hillsdale, NJ: Lawrence Erlbaum Associates; 1994.
18. Beebe B, Lachman F. Infant research and adult treatment: Co-constructing Interactions. Hillsdale, NJ: Analytic Press; 2005.
19. Bateman AW, Fonagy P. Handbook of mentalizing in mental health practice. Arlington, VA: American Psychiatric Publishing; 2012.
20. Mahler M, Pine F. The Birth of the Human Infant. New York: Basic Books; 1975.
21. Blatt SJ, Levy KN. Attachment theory, psychoanalysis, personality development and psychopathology. Psychoanal Inq 2003;23:102–50.
22. Main M, Hesse E. Parents' unresolved traumatic experiences are related to infant disorganized attachment status: Is frightened or frightening parental behavior the linking mechanism? In: Greenberg MT, Cicchetti D, Cummings EM, editors. Attachment in the preschool years (pp. 161–182). Chicago, IL: University of Chicago Press; 1990.
23. Main M, Solomon J. Procedures for identifying infants as disorganized/disoriented during the Ainsworth strange situation. In: Greenberg MT, Cicchetti D, Cummings EM, editors. Attachment in the preschool years (pp. 121–160). Chicago, IL: University of Chicago Press; 1990.
24. Main M. The organized categories of infant, child, and adult attachment: Flexible vs. inflexible attention under attachment-related stress. J Am Psychoanal Assoc 2000;48:1055–96.
25. Bowlby J. Attachment and Loss, Vol. 1, 2nd edition. New York: Basic Books; 1983.
26. Ainsworth MDS, Blehar M, Waters E, et al. Patterns of Attachment. Hillsdale, NJ: Erlbaum; 1978.
27. Lieberman AF, Van Horn P. "Don't hit my mommy!": a manual for child-parent psychotherapy for young witness of family violence. Washington, DC: Zero to Three; 2005.
28. Fraiberg S. Clinical Studies in infant mental health. New York: Basic Books; 1980.
29. Freud A. Normality and pathology in childhood. The writings of Anna Freud, Vol. 6. New York: International University Press; 1965.
30. Freud S. Three essays on the Theory of Sexuality, Standard Edition, Vol. 7. London: The Hogart Press and the Institute of Psycho-Analysis; 1905.
31. Toth SL, Rogosch FA, Manly JT, et al. The efficacy of toddler-parent psychotherapy to reorganize attachment in the young offspring of mothers with major depressive disorder: a randomized preventive trial. J Consult Clin Psychol 2006;74:1006–16.
32. Slade A. Parental reflective functioning: an introduction. Attach Hum Dev 2005; 7(3):269–81.
33. Bowlby J. A Secure Base: Clinical Applications of Attachment Theory. London: Routledge; 1988.
34. Steele H, Steele M. On the origins of reflective functioning. In: Busch F, editor. Mentalization: theoretical considerations, research findings and clinical implications. New York: Analytic Press; 2008. p. 133–56.
35. Strathearn L, Fonagy P, Amico J, et al. Adult attachment predicts maternal brain & oxytocin response to infant cues. Neuropsychopharmacology 2001;34: 2655–66.

36. Ainsworth MDS. Infancy in Uganda: Infant care and the growth of love. Baltimore, MD: The Johns Hopkins University Press; 1967.
37. Carlson EA, Sroufe LA. Contributions of attachment theory to developmental psychopathology. In: Cichetti D, Cohen DJ, editors. Developmental psychopathology: theory and methods, vol. 1. New York: Wiley; 1995. p. 581–617.
38. Van Ijzendoorn M. Adult attachment representations, parental responsiveness and infant attachment. A meta-analysis on the predictive validity of the AAI. Psychol Bull 1995;117(3):387–403.
39. Fonagy P, Steele M, Steele H, et al. Attachment, the reflective self and borderline states: the predictive specificity of the attachment adult interview and pathological emotional development. In: Goldberg S, Mueir R, Kerr J, editors. Attachment theory: social, developmental and clinical perspectives. Hillside (NJ): Analytic Press; 1995. p. 233–79.
40. Beebe B, Lachmann F. The relational turn in psychoanalysis: a dyadic systems view from infant research. Contemp Psychoanal 2003;39(3).
41. Siegel DJ. Toward an interpersonal neurobiology of the developing mind: attachment relationships, "mindsight" and neural integration. Infant Ment Health J 2001; 22(1–2):67–94.
42. Strathearn L, Fonagy P, Amico J, et al. Adult attachment maternal brain and oxytocin response to infant cues. Neuropsychopharmacology 2009;34: 2655–66.
43. National Scientific Council on the Developing Child (2008). Mental problems in early childhood can impair learning and behavior for life. Working paper No. 6. Available at: http://developingchild.harvard.edu/index.php/resources/reports_and_working_papers/working_papers/wp6/. Accessed October 6, 2012.
44. Fonagy P, Target M. Who is help by child psychoanalysis? A sample study of disruptive children, from the anna freud centre retrospective investigation. Bul Anna Freud Centre 1994;17:291–315.
45. Heinicke CM, Ramsey-Klee DM. Outcome of child psychotherapy as a function of frequency of session. Journal of the American Academy of Psychiatry 1986;25(2): 247–53.
46. Moran GS, Fonagy P, Kurtz A, et al. A controlled study of the psychoanalytic treatment of brittle diabetes. Journal of the American Academy of Child and Adolescent Psychiatry 1991;30:241–57.
47. Roth A, Fonagy P. What works for whom?: a critical review of psychotherapy research. London: The Guildford Press; 1996.
48. Malberg NT. Thinking and feeling in the context of chronic illness: a mentalization-based group intervention with adolescents. In: Midgley N, Vrouva I, editors. Minding the child: mentalization-based interventions with children, young people and their families. (United Kingdom): Routledge; 2012. p. 147–62.
49. Novick J, Kelly Novick K. Working with parents makes therapy work. New York: Jason Aronson; 2005.
50. Rossouw T. Self-harm in young people: is MBT the answer?. In: Midgley N, Vrouva I, editors. Minding the child: mentalization-based interventions with children, young people and their families. (United Kingdom): Routledge; 2012. p. 131–44.
51. Freud A. Nursery school and child guidance clinic, Interactions between. The Writings of Anna Freud, Vol. 5. New York: Int Univ Press; 1966 [1965]. p. 369–78.
52. Shonkoff JP, Phillips D, editors. From neurons to neighborhoods: the science of early childhood development. Committee on integrating the science of early childhood development. Washington, DC: National Academy Press; 2000.

53. Suchman NE, DeCoste C, Castiglioni N, et al. The Mothers and Toddlers Program: Preliminary findings from an attachment-based parenting intervention for substance abusing mothers. Psychoanalytic Psychology 2008;25:499–517.
54. Twemlow SW, Fonagy P, Sacco FC. A developmental approach to mentalizing communities: a model for social change. Bull Menninger Clin 2005;69(4):265–81.
55. Twemlow SW, Sacco FC, Hough G. A socio-psychoanalytic perspective of group dynamics, cults and terrorism I: the context of terrorism. Soc Anim 2003;5:57–78.
56. Allen JG, Fonagy P, Bateman A. Mentalizing in clinical practice. Arlington, VA: American Psychiatric Publishing, Inc; 2008.
57. Malberg NT, Fonagy P, Mayes L. Contemporary psychoanalysis in a pediatric hemodialysis unit: development of a mentalization-based group intervention for adolescent patients with end-stage renal disease. The annual of psychoanalysis, vol. XXXVI–XXXVII. Catskill (New York): Mental Health Resources; 2009. 2008–2009.

Treating Childhood Trauma

Lenore C. Terr, MD

KEYWORDS

• Childhood PTSD • Abreaction • Context • Correction • Memory of trauma
• Attachment and trauma • Trauma and development • Mixing treatment techniques

KEY POINTS

When treating childhood trauma psychodynamically, the therapist must keep several points in mind:

- Trauma "looks" different to each young person and it varies over each stage of development.
- Trauma sets up life themes.
- Traumatic memory is malleable and may change over time through familial talk, therapeutic work, suggestion, outside manipulation, and life experience.
- Three principles of healing are extremely useful in helping traumatized children in psychotherapy: abreaction (emotional expression), context (cognitive understanding), and correction (behavioral or fantasized change).
- Attachment problems may outweigh traumatic experiences in young individuals.
- One can fluidly mix psychoanalytically derived psychotherapy, play therapy, cognitive-behavioral therapy, counseling, and medication for childhood trauma.

INTRODUCTION

Childhood trauma is a comparatively new disorder to the fields of psychiatry, psychoanalysis, and mental health. Early in his career, Sigmund Freud lost interest in questions concerning "utter helplessness" in the face of external events, turning instead to explorations of the internal worlds of adults and children. His daughter Anna, a great observer of the inner lives of children, noted how an English lad, named "Bertie," exhibited terror of the World War II bombings through his play.[1] But she did not go on to fully characterize the posttraumatic condition from which he was suffering.

In 1976, when a Chowchilla school bus carrying 26 children, ages 5 to 14, was kidnapped and the children were buried alive (eventually to rescue themselves after 27 hours), the condition "childhood trauma" was studied within a few months and fully described.[2] Four to 5 years after the kidnapping, a long-term study was accomplished[3] and a comparison group from similar towns miles away was also interviewed

Department of Psychiatry, Langley Porter Institute, University of California San Francisco School of Medicine, 401 Parnassus Avenue, San Francisco, CA 94143, USA
E-mail address: scott.terrmd@sbcglobal.net

Child Adolesc Psychiatric Clin N Am 22 (2013) 51–66
http://dx.doi.org/10.1016/j.chc.2012.08.003 childpsych.theclinics.com
1056-4993/13/$ – see front matter

and assessed.[4] Since then, other studies of groups of children exposed to a certain single event have offered additional answers to the question: "What is childhood trauma?"[5]

WHAT IS CHILDHOOD TRAUMA?

The childhood trauma problem is more complicated than the effects of single events, however. Young people are often prone to repeated assaults, sexual misuses, neglect, and mistreatment.[6–8] And even if only one event occurs, as in the field studies noted previously, the results may be complicated. A sibling or a parent may die, for instance, and thus the child's attachments may be drastically disrupted.[9,10] A young person might be injured or disfigured, leading to repeated surgeries, bullying at school, and chronic pain. Poverty, a divorce, a pending lawsuit, or parental naiveté may prevent the youngster from seeing a professional for years. These complications lead to more chronic and complex traumas than were observed at Chowchilla.

In children, traumatic complexities frequently lead to such problems as ongoing depressions, numbing of emotions, character changes, and aggressive, destructive behaviors.[11] I call the simple traumas "Type I" and the complicated ones "Type II," saving room for a number of conditions that I call "Crossovers." Crossovers carry characteristics engendered by a single situation that creates long-term, ongoing insults to the child's development. Other investigators refer to Type II trauma and Crossovers as "complex" posttraumatic stress disorder (PTSD).[12] No matter what terminology one chooses, however, it is clear that complicated traumas are harder to treat than single-blow conditions. It often becomes difficult to determine the correct diagnosis for a complicated trauma in a latency-age child or an adolescent. Is it "complex trauma" (PTSD) or a biologic entity, such as major depressive disorder? Is it a personality disorder or an attachment disorder? One basic point, however, remains clear. If trauma is part of the child's life experience, no matter what diagnosis is ultimately chosen, the trauma must become part of the child's treatment.

DIAGNOSING CHILDHOOD TRAUMA

Defining Traumatic Events

When asked, children describe the fears they experienced during traumatic events differently from the way adults do. For instance, fears of death and physical injury (threats that characterize most adult traumas) are not necessarily the strongest fears on children's lists. Most children younger than 5 do not understand the completeness of death. A highly religious older child or adolescent may not make a sharp distinction between dying on earth and living in heaven. As for injuries, children's lack of knowledge and experience does not fully enable them to assess what physical harm may lurk in their own activities or the activities that others impose on them. On the other hand, some children readily catch on to the feelings of dehumanization and humiliation connected with some traumas. Those situations may qualify for such youngsters as traumatic, whereas others do not see it the same way. An almost universal childhood fear inspired by terrible events is the dread of being cut off from caregiver(s) and what is known as "home." Young people are profoundly aware of their helplessness without parents. The father or mother, if an abuser, is often safe from accusation by their child, not only because of the child's sense of shame in telling anyone about attacks from a parent, but because of the potential loss of care, food, shelter, or the noninjuring parent. No matter how much the physical or sexual abuses may have hurt, confused, and humiliated the child, the loss of primary attachment is frequently conceived by a youngster as worse.

CLINICAL CASE: CHILD ABUSE BY PARENT

An 11-year-old girl was reported by her teacher to have been sexually abused by her stepfather. A gynecologic examination at a nearby hospital confirmed the teacher's report. A criminal trial was set, according to the newspapers reporting the crime, but the girl refused to testify against her stepdad. The judge hearing the case placed the child in jail for contempt of court. She remained there all through the summer. Still refusing to testify, she was finally released to enter middle school and, theoretically, to experience more sex abuse at home. Her unprosecuted, undivorced stepparent was the sole wage earner of her family. Hopefully, the child protection agency in her community insisted on establishing a treatment program for her and all others concerned. But one wonders....

Not only is the loss of attachment a profound worry for a child, but fears of being exposed in public, bullied, or isolated by peers sometimes achieve the stature of trauma. Some examples are the demeaning ones (ie, a boy was unknowingly filmed and then broadcast by a roommate having sex with another male), or the incessantly repeated ones (ie, a mildly autistic boy is called "germy" and not allowed within 3 feet of anyone in his classroom), or the unusually violent ones (ie, a high school girl is attacked in a gym shower with shampoo bottles by 3 classmates). Witnessing a terrible event also qualifies as a trauma in certain instances.[13] It depends on what was witnessed, where the witness was, what the victim's relationship was to the witness, how much personal responsibility the witness took, and what the young witness thought was actually happening.[5,14]

In summary, a trauma is not only defined by the type of outside incident that causes it, but by the meaning the child or adolescent affixes to it. How the mental condition is manifest comes directly from that meaning.[13]

Obtaining the Full Story and the Full Symptomatology

A childhood trauma evaluation includes reviewing all pertinent records, including court material; interviewing family members; reading newspaper accounts if available; and speaking to any involved professionals, such as teachers, pediatricians, police, and the child's attorney. If there is a question of head injury, a neurologist and/or neuropsychologist should be considered. The child is asked for his or her own account. The evaluating clinician's questioning should be done as broadly and nondirectively as possible: "Tell me all about the accident," or "Can you describe what happened to you? I need to hear the whole story," or "The police brought you here to talk to me. What was it all about? You can begin anywhere you'd like and I'll just listen."

It usually takes more than one 45-minute appointment with the child or adolescent to get a whole trauma story, especially if one is trying to hear all of its attendant emotions and thoughts. It also takes time to review the entire gamut of the child's symptoms. These include all repetitions, even those, such as play or reenactments, that the child does not realize are connected to the event. (One asks: "Have you done anything weird, or done something that got you in trouble?" or "What kind of pretend stuff and games have you been playing?" Then one waits for the patient to tell all about it.) Other important symptoms are trauma-specific and generalized fears. One must look for indications of emotional, cognitive, or physical turn-offs and numbings. Importantly, one must check for the child's concerns about trusting others, and a lack of faith in the future. It usually takes a few sessions with the child to obtain all of this.

Constructing a Formulation

In a trauma evaluation, the formulation will include the type and nature of the event, the nature of the child's current and/or future support systems, and the child's current and

CLINICAL CASE: "LIFE THEME" VARIANCE

Two adult brothers attended a sexually abusive day care program for preschoolers. Groups of children were engaged in sex with each other, often with an adult participating, as well. The brothers were there in different years because of their distant spacing at birth. The oldest brother "forgot" all about the multiple abuses until some vague shards of memory returned to him when he was fully grown. But he had symptoms all along. The younger one "knew" the details of this abuse throughout his childhood, but could not speak about it or take action at the time. The older boy, an attorney today, has lived out a lifelong theme of combating corruption, be it in private or institutional acts. He also sees himself as a helper to females, especially those in sexually based distress. The younger boy, on the other hand, an anesthesiologist, wishes to disappear. He lives out his life with aims to do good, but to do it secretly. He lives without women (or men) in his personal sphere and he sculpts beautiful abstract art in his spare time. Each brother has fashioned a life theme from his traumatic preschool days. But each theme is quite different, despite the similarity of the trauma.

future developmental stages. (For example, if a child was thrown against a wall at age 2, will the child become more violent in adolescence?) For each stage, a different interpretation or meaning may have become attached to the mental representation of the trauma. If this special meaning is known, it should be included in the formulation. What a child thinks and feels about an event becomes the guideline for the treatment plan. What "life theme" the trauma imposes on the growing child is of great importance.

TREATING TRAUMA USING 3 BASIC PRINCIPLES

1. Abreaction
2. Context
3. Correction

Abreaction

Abreaction is the patient's full and complete expression of emotions connected to the trauma.[15] Traumatic events make children angry, horrified, scared, overexcited, sad, and confused. Sometime these feelings are so mixed that a youngster, even an older one, cannot put words to the amalgam. Sometimes a child has never learned the words for the emotions. The child must learn them now. In some cases, the clinician must teach these words through little games or picture books depicting emotions, or must ask the child's parent or teachers to show the child the words. They can be taught with regard to a fairy tale, for instance. "How does Goldilocks feel?" "How would it feel to be Little Red Riding Hood?" "When Jack met the Giant, what was in Jack's heart?" "What was in Mr. Giant's heart?" For children who don't respond to old stories, the "here and now" works, too. "Who cried at preschool today?" "What do you think she was feeling?" "Do you ever cry? Tell me the kinds of things that make you cry."

Abreaction was one of the first techniques used psychiatrically to help children with their traumatic experiences. David Levy, a distinguished American child psychiatrist and psychoanalyst of the mid-twentieth century, wrote about using behavioral abreaction to combat the anxieties connected with unexplained tonsillectomies and other such medical procedures. Children came into Dr Levy's office and aggressively squeezed clay, pounded toys, and otherwise shouted and played away their wild emotions following surprising and bad hospital experiences.[16] In child psychoanalysis and psychotherapy, the abreactive technique of Levy gradually faded away. His writings, however, inspired a new age of humane pediatric care. He had made 3 very

CLINICAL CASE: ABREACTION

When I met her, this 7-year-old girl was refusing all visitations with her mother because of a long history of maternal attacks, giving her a burn, a number of bad bruises, and a broken clavicle. The little girl flitted about my office, buzzing me and my furniture with a swarm of airplanes, spacecraft, and flying monsters. The noise, the sudden lunges of aircraft, and the crash landings on my desk simulated the old attacks from a mother whom she had not been allowed to see for months. But more important than mere simulation, the aircraft and damaging reptiles were expressing to me this little girl's fears and furies. They were showing me metaphorically what she had experienced, while bringing her a modicum of relief.

important points. Children should be told what's going to happen to them. Their parents should be with them through hospitalizations. And, most important to this discussion, expressing previously unexpressed feelings greatly helps traumatized children.

Currently, traumatized children are asked by psychotherapists to tell their stories again, this time with feeling. They also can play out their emotions, using such devices as dinosaurs, armies, doll houses, and even rap songs. It is rare for abreaction to be the only avenue used, however, because context and correction are so helpful. A full and complete treatment of trauma, using abreaction alone, is hard to envision today.

Biochemical and functional imaging studies have shown that the amygdala, a structure within each temporal lobe, is an important site for emotional memory[17] and for reactivity to threat.[18] When terrifying memories are reintroduced and reviewed, through purposely thinking about an old trauma, the amygdalar memories apparently become reactivated. At such moments, these memories may be more amenable to reconsideration and reorganization. Taking this newly discovered biologic factor into account, one can postulate that the old-fashioned technique of abreactively treating a child's trauma, be it in splashes of paint or in splashes of tears, helps its eventual containment and, perhaps, its defeat.

Context

Context is the child's understanding, clarification, and perspective on a trauma. If the child comes to see a terrible experience more historically, geographically, rhythmically, poetically, scientifically, the child will benefit.[19] Context is primarily a cognitive process. Because children experience traumas at various ages, the context offered

CLINICAL CASE: CONTEXT

The 2-year-old sister of a 5-year-old kindergarten boy suddenly ran out into the street from the suburban front yard where they were playing. She was hit and run over by a motorcycle. After a hospitalization, she recovered without sequelae. The kindergartener, however, developed the idea that he had been entirely responsible. He was traumatized by what he saw. When, at age 6, he was brought for psychiatric treatment, he fretted that if he had been nicer, more engaged in their play, more "something," the accident would not have happened. In his psychotherapy, he needed to rethink how toddlers behave. He had to reconsider his sister's very sudden move, her unawareness of the danger, her naiveté to cars and motorcycles. Then, too, weren't there adult responsibilities, as well—the motorcycle driver? The builder who was constructing a picket fence around the yard, but hadn't yet finished? His parents who had let the toddler out unsupervised? The young witness was just a witness—he certainly was not the creator of his little sister's miseries. The boy needed more than a year of sessions to become asymptomatic. Part of the problem had been his parents' tendency to blame him.

them in psychotherapy must be geared specifically to their age and stage of development. Likely, the youngster has already spontaneously developed his or her own contexts to the trauma in the minutes to years before anyone took the child to a mental health professional. Some of these personalized meanings, including "omens"[20] or "cognitive reappraisals,"[21] may sound bizarre. It is difficult to rework these very personal, and often mistaken, contexts. But they must be tackled and revised in psychotherapy, be it in play, talk, or both.

Correction

Correction is the act of finding a behavioral or fantasized way of turning a trauma around. It may be altruistic, preventive, personally triumphant, or even a bit revengeful; but it must feel "right" to the particular child. Children are able to correct for their traumas in their actions or in fantasy (play, drawings, stories).[22] These behavioral solutions are a very effective part of the dynamic psychotherapy of trauma. Even if a trauma is absolutely uncorrectable—say, someone close to the child was killed—it still can be therapeutically corrected, in part, by looking to the future with the child, or in considering what might be done in our country (such as building a safer highway) or less-developed countries, or as a new proposed law. One likes to see hurt children become altruistic about other children. As they grow older, one likes to see them learn to babysit (with supervision in graduated amounts). To start, traumatized children can take responsibility for pets, learn to cook and feed others, bring treats to class at school, and post on-line pictures of younger relatives or friends. Learning to drive is often a healing experience for traumatized teenagers, eventually giving them control over a large, dangerous device. It is often helpful to take a long time—a couple of years, perhaps—to go through the training process, including a few private lessons at a driving school. Yes, these are "behavioral" treatments, but they mix in very well with the psychodynamic psychotherapies.

Obviously, any correction that is meaningful must be geared to the particular nature of the child's trauma and the child's age, stage, and mental/physical abilities. It may require more help than the psychotherapist can carry out alone. In managing the behaviors that are so often part of correction, the clinician will frequently have to deal with a teacher, a school principal, a doctor, even a driving instructor. Parents, of course are the main assisters, and sometimes they can perform correction as a kind of "filial therapy."[23,24]

CLINICAL CASE: CORRECTION

A 2.5-year-old girl had been fully toilet trained and quite grown up when she suddenly regressed. Her nursery school called home to ask about it. The same situation had sprung up at home. When this little girl was an infant, her mother had almost died of cancer. She fully recovered through radiation and chemotherapy. Most likely this child had overheard something or had been told something terrifying about the cancer right now, well after the fact, at age 32 months. It must have been highly threatening to her 2-year-old sense of attachment and autonomy. When she came to my office, I included the little girl's mother in our appointment and the child chose to play "Princess." Everything Princess did had to be very, very grown up, we all determined together. This was a correction to the child's behavior and it proved long-lasting. But her mother, as we decided in advance, also explained to the child at home what her illness had originally been and when (2 years before) the doctors had told her that she was cured. I saw the child in my office waiting room again when she was 4. Her regression—after that one, single meeting—had not happened again. Correction had been the largest element to her recovery, but context and abreaction had also played their parts, particularly in her "talk" with her mother.

THREE POTENTIAL COMPLICATIONS TO TRAUMA TREATMENT

1. Memory
2. Attachment
3. Transference and Countertransference

Memory Work

Once in a while, a child's old shards of remembrance, or the child's drawings, and/or the child's repeated play can be put together with what is already known about the child's life to construct a kind of "story" of the child's trauma. This can be helpful to the child and family. However, I write here of memory work, or "reconstruction" as it is sometimes called, mainly to discourage its general use. Traumatic memory is a highly controversial subject today because of concerns about "suggestion."[25,26] A child's memory of trauma can be influenced by peers, family, TV shows, the Internet, police questioning, and any number of other outside forces, but it can also be influenced through the youngster's psychotherapy. Our field's influence over memory became so harshly criticized by the broadcasters, magazines, and newspapers of the late 1990s that an attack against the whole idea of psychotherapy ensued. Luckily, the field survived as evidenced in small part by the articles in this collection of *Child and Adolescent Psychiatric Clinics of North America*.

It is important to keep in mind that reconstructive memory work is not necessary to the treatment of childhood trauma. Youngsters show their memories in what they say, what they feel, and what they do.[27,28] The child's story, as far as it is known, even if fragmented, is the story that the clinician will work with. If there are hospital records or police reports, these can be taken as pieces of real information to be shared with the young patient when he or she is ready. If there was an eyewitness, that person's statement can also be shared. The idea is to guess less and to know more.

A newspaper account can be searched for, and if available, can be used in the youngster's treatment. A trauma "scene" can be visited by the child and family again; or it can be mapped or drawn by the child in the doctor's office. What the child's parents know of the event can be related to the child, at home perhaps after counseling, or in the psychiatric consultation room. What is important is to avoid suggestion and to let the child lead the way.

Direct attempts to elicit "forgotten" trauma stories, through such techniques as hypnotism, sodium amytal administration, eye movement desensitization, or "anatomically correct" dolls,[29] must be used with great caution, if at all. The therapist's inadvertent tendencies to suggest and the patient's wishes to cooperate may create more serious problems than they relieve.

Patients and clients need not strain to remember. Working in the "here and now" and using the techniques discussed in this article are usually good enough to relieve the child. The younger the child, the more suggestible he or she is. Because of the intensity of the psychotherapeutic relationship, however, a patient of any age may pick up a doctor's suggestion and internalize it.

I will offer a short personal example here. About 10 years ago, I gave a lecture on memory to a large professional audience. In it, I spoke of my earliest remembrance, a fluttering shadow coming down on my face from above. It was a frightening memory, and when I was still a child I asked my mother about it. She remembered. She said she had been walking me in Prospect Park, Brooklyn, in my baby carriage when a pigeon landed on the hood, terrifying me (I left New York when I was 11 months old). I used this example to show the audience at my talk that you may need a second witness to explain an infantile memory. One of the audience members came to me afterward to ask a question. "How do you know that the fluttering shadow wasn't really your father's penis and that your mother was covering for him?" This represented the extreme of what memory reconstruction, if administered thoughtlessly, can do. With traumatized children, we cannot implant such ideas just because we might find them interesting or intellectually challenging. Remember, "First, do no harm." (Parenthetically, my memory of the pigeon was not influenced by the audience member's suggestion.)

Attachment

Many times a therapist must work long and hard with a young patient who has suffered traumatic loss, or broken relationships, abandonments, foster care, institutional living, and other threats to important relationships, which are often associated with trauma (abuse, neglect, and on-off connectedness). Although the attachment issues are usually seen as primary and the trauma, secondary, do not forget to treat the trauma. Abreaction, context, and correction can be used in concert with the other techniques that are aimed at grief, loss, and neglect. Several other topics in this issue offer suggestions for dealing with such problems, among them see the article by Midgley and the article by Shapiro elsewhere in the issue. And so I will leave the subject, while reiterating how central it is to any child's well-being.

Transference and Countertransference

With traumatized children who suffered single uncomplicated events, such as an accident, a natural disaster, an assault by a stranger, transference does not usually arise as an important issue. The therapist is seen as a "nice" or "good" person who will be helpful. The child almost automatically trusts the doctor. If the single event, however, was accompanied by painful procedures in a hospital or a surgical suite, then it is highly important for the psychiatrist to establish that he is a "talking doctor" and will not be giving any shots or physicals. If the therapist has an obligation to file a report, the therapist must say so. If the therapist will be visiting school about the trauma, the therapist must be frank. When a youngster has an injury or a wound and wants to show it to the therapist, it is reasonable to look at it without touching. It is even more reasonable to have a parent or an office assistant present while one looks.

Transference becomes a larger issue when a child has been abused by one or more caretakers. Now, the "good" doctor is not to be trusted because other people, seemingly "good," betrayed the child. Sexually or physically abused children may act angry

CASE EXAMPLES: TRANSFERENCE

At a therapeutic school where adolescents who haven't been able to function in the public schools attend for a year or two, a number of students automatically show negative transference to the consulting psychiatrist. One 13-year-old boy from a family of drug users (a jailed mother lost her parental rights long ago) insists on reading the doctor's notes and knowing where the notes will be going (to the school's and the doctor's file) before walking out in a huff. The doctor tells him pleasantly she'll see him again soon. (He seeks her out the next time she is there.) A 14-year-old boy tells the same doctor about 4 recent physical abuses that never happened (lies). The truth is that as a young boy he was repeatedly physically abused, but not now. His teacher begins working with him about lying. He will see the doctor later. A 16-year-old girl who lives alone with her quiet, negligent father (her mother is in state prison) assumes total silence with the doctor the first time they meet. Then, 2 weeks later, she opens up and tells her doctor quite a bit, especially her most recent concerns about sex, birth control, and her future.

all the time. They may be withdrawn. Or they may be seductive, coyly manipulative, and "hail-fellow-well-met." On getting to know them better, they are often unemotional and uncaring. Such children do not ordinarily accept verbal therapeutic interpretations of this kind of transferential behavior. Instead, they may eventually accept the proofs inherent in their therapies—slowly given. One gradually proves that therapists can be trusted.[30] Unattached, multiply wounded children often respond to mutual interests with their psychotherapists—enjoyment of a type of music, or a sport, or a gadget, for instance. Talking or playing together without much "meat" to the conversation is a good way of breaking past such transferential blockades. In other words, small talk is not a waste of time with a repeatedly traumatized child or adolescent.

Countertransference operates from the very beginning of work with traumatized children. Their stories are horrifying. In eliciting the full story "with feelings," the clinician may feel overwhelmed. Children's true tales crash through our shields of invincibility. A therapist may temporarily experience pains, anxiety, even phobias or depression. Occupational "burn out" is common.

A few suggestions may help:

1. Talking with other professionals, especially those working with other traumatized young people, can be useful. One good friend and colleague also working in the field of trauma is usually enough. The talks should happen whenever needed and recur relatively frequently.
2. Occasional consultations about trauma cases with a senior psychotherapist outside one's own institution can buttress one's morale. Even if this involves some financial sacrifice, it is an educational opportunity and can enable a modicum of emotional release.
3. In scheduling, if you have a wide-ranging practice, try not to place appointments with traumatized children in large clumps. Spreading out the timing helps.
4. Do research. If simply for your own numerical counts (or if one is involved in a large cooperative institutional effort), doing research preserves your interest in trauma beyond the single case. It aids your sense of self-esteem and your longevity in the field.
5. Get away totally. Use weekend days to look at a mountain, swim in a lake, fish in a stream, tend your garden. Release your mind. Small talk, the newspaper, your iPod, a good book—all of these are remedies to the pains of treating trauma. There are bigger things and tinier things in the world that offer you a sense of balance.
6. Keep your friends and family close.
7. Write.
8. Teach.

TREATMENT MODALITIES

Talk Therapy

Traumatized children and adolescents need to feel good coming away from their therapy sessions. It is important to make the treatment feel relatively pleasant, even though very unpleasant events must be discussed in detail. This is in contrast to some of the other psychodynamic therapies, particularly those aimed at adults. Although some adult treatments set up frustrating silences or nonresponsive echoings from the therapist, traumatized children do not do well under these conditions. These kids have experienced so much pain and loneliness in their lives that their therapy sessions must present a contrast. The talk moves back and forth, a fluid dialogue. The therapist says what he or she thinks is a true answer to the child's question. Talk is straight. It flows.

The aim of talk therapy for trauma is to encourage the 3 healing expressions noted earlier in this article: abreaction, context, and correction. The conversation between doctor and patient, however, may have more to do with the "here-and-now" in the child's life than it does with the old traumatic events. How the old trauma influences the present situation is pointed out whenever it is clear. Little exercises in the behavioral mode of therapy are offered, if they are appropriate. Grades can be offered—an A+ for instance, for a new mode of relating that a child has not attempted before. "High-5s" and "shout outs" are encouragements well within the realm of a satisfying session. The idea is to have a little fun while discussing what—up to now—has not been a fun-filled stay on earth.

Much of the "talk" is playful in good talk therapy for trauma. Jokes—if not on the child—are great. Word games, bets, codes, magic are to be encouraged. One is trying to let the hurt child sense that some hurts can be looked at from a great distance, or turned around into their opposites. Some "talk" in talk therapies for trauma can be devoted to practice scenarios—teaching a child, for instance, how to make an emergency phone call and then practicing the calls; showing a child how to barricade a door, how to confront a perpetrator, how to tell a school administrator something important. Much can also be accomplished by playing with ideas about superheroes, sports heroes, princesses, cowboys, singers, stars. "What would Batman do?" is a terrific question, if the child likes Batman (after all, he was traumatized, too).[31] In more contemporary language, a young baseball player like Buster Posey, who was so badly injured that many people thought he'd never come back, makes a nucleus for lots of talk. A new movie—if the therapist saw it, too—or a popular icon, like Harry Potter, can be enormously helpful. In May 2012 the former basketball star, Shaquille O'Neal, got his doctorate degree in education. One can have fun—and inspire the right kid—with "yack" about "Dr Shaq."

All talk therapy, in other words, does not have to be pithy. With a traumatized child or adolescent, the talk should be, at least in part, playful. The mutual storytelling technique[32,33] is extremely useful in this regard. The clinician can start the tale—"Once there was a boy, named Jake, who lived in Alabama and—" and then the client or patient can be encouraged to join in. From there on, the adult and child can construct a metaphoric tale, encompassing abreactions, contexts, and corrections galore. With young people, these metaphors work just as powerfully as direct talk. And frequently, they are less threatening to the patient.

CLINICAL CASE: TALK THERAPY

An 18-year-old college student was raped and threatened with imminent death on a date. She did not realize how badly she was injured until a week later when a doctor photographed her wounds. Too frightened to press criminal charges, she saw a psychiatrist, but told her she was coming for attention-deficit/hyperactivity disorder, which actually had been a longstanding problem. It was 5 months after the rape. She had not described the attack yet to her parents. The rapist was attempting to "get together" again. This young patient was operating on denial.

The girl's talk therapy—not many appointments because of the distance of her university—centered on scenario making. She needed to tell the rapist what she thought and felt about him. Could she practice it now? She needed to learn to say the word, "rape." Could she make herself intone the word? She needed to thoroughly express her sense of robbery of her personal rights. She also needed to understand the difference between this very troubled young man and a new boyfriend she was beginning to see. All of this—both playful (the scenarios) and pithy (about the new boyfriend) could be handled through therapeutic talk. It included abreaction, context, and correction.

Play Therapy

Play and art work are extremely expressive and successful ways to psychodynamically treat traumatized children. Almost anything in the office a traumatized youngster picks up might be considered an object of play. One child rubbed sofa cushions together, simulating incestuous sex. A different child drew pictures of an isolated monkey to depict her own sense of being cut off from her parents while experiencing sex with a pedophile.

I keep some of my office toys out in the open and others, in cabinets. If a child seems interested in playing, I show the child what I have. What is so interesting about posttraumatic play is that it is so inevitable.[34] The grim-looking trauma victim, no matter how young, is bound and determined to play. At ages in the youngest and oldest (late adolescence) ranges of childhood, these kids often prefer play to talk. Their play is very thinly disguised. They love stories, like "Little Red Riding Hood" or "The Three Bears," because these tales so closely simulate the sensations of trauma. The wicked witch or the toothy dinosaur is an object of choice for a child who previously has been robbed of all choice.

The therapist enters the child's play directly, picking up a dinosaur or Red Riding Hood's wolf. The therapist takes the child's instructions as to which object to "be"; or throws in his or her own inventive idea to add to the child's play. The plan is to use therapeutic play to effect abreaction, context, or correction in the child. Not all 3 can usually occur at once. But frequently play will allow at least one of these to be dealt with. "Is Cowboy scared?" "Might Cowboy meet with other cowboys and make a strategy to defeat the dinos?" "What can we do about the other injured cowboys? Should we build a hospital?" Some of the play can be psychoanalytically based,[35,36] some can happen in a Jungian sand tray,[37] some can be cognitive-behavioral,[38] and some can take a mixed approach.[39]

When playing with traumatized toddlers, preschoolers, and school-age children, one has the option to include parents and/or siblings in the session.[40] When a parent barely understands the child's problem or needs to learn how to play with the youngster, this

CLINICAL CASE: PLAY THERAPY

A 6-year-old boy, swimming in the ocean, was suddenly swept out to sea by a wicked riptide. Luckily, his father, an expert swimmer, was able to rescue and resuscitate him. The boy was almost immediately taken to a psychiatrist who expertly played with him on themes around learning to swim, facing the ocean, and trusting to separate from his father. He drew pictures of sea monsters and then wiped them out with black marking pens. He flopped dolls about the floor and enunciated their "sinking" feelings. He learned that you could check out the tides by phoning a certain number. After a year, he stopped therapy, greatly improved.

Then at 12, in middle school, he developed a fear of toilets. He jumped if one automatically flushed. He refused to sit on one. His family found a new therapist who told him they could play "toilet" together. They would visit the various Men's Rooms in the doctor's office building and even sneak into a Ladies Room or two (if no one was there). After a couple sessions of checking out all the automatic toilet mechanisms and seeing how they worked (a kind of play for a scientifically curious boy of 12), the boy and his doctor had an insight. He was afraid of the suction! If he fell into a toilet, it would—just like the riptide—suck him out to sea. They went to the building bathrooms to play once more, this time checking out the sizes of the toilet outlets. "No way!" The boy was absolutely safe, he realized. This ended his second round of treatment. The first time he was treated, he had psychodynamic play therapy. The second time, he had a mix of cognitive-behavioral treatment and psychodynamic treatment. Both worked.

can be of great help.[41] It can also help if one plans to have the parent buttress the child's treatment with filial sessions at home. If a parent is present, the psychiatrist can exercise other options—to ask the parent and the child to play as he or she watches, or to play while the parent observes, or to all join in the play together. These are not, however, ways to "cure" abusive parents. If abuse is ongoing, all the talk and play in the world may easily have no effect. Such parents often need their own private sessions to "exorcize" their own personal "ghosts."[42] Sometimes they must be removed from their children altogether.

Parental (or Caretaker) Counseling

With traumatized children, parents and/or caretakers need guidance. Special sessions can be set up for the parents. Or 5 to 10 minutes can be carved out from each of the child's sessions for parental counseling. The therapist has options as to the timings of the carve-outs. If parents come first, the clinician gets to hear what happened this week. This is helpful when a child is not forthcoming. But the young person may see an early carve-out as an unhelpful form of parental "tattling." If the carve-out comes after the child's session, the young patient may consider it as evidence of a breach in doctor-patient confidentiality. The psychiatrist must explain that he is giving a general run-down of what is going on and advice to parents, not anything specific about what the child said or did in therapy. Many times I let a child be present at the end of the session to hear what we are discussing and to throw in suggestions or objections. These therapeutic decisions about timings are usually spontaneous. No specific routine need be enforced.

If a trauma involves deep grief and mourning in a family, or if a parent is suffering from trauma as well, it is often helpful to involve another family member (an aunt, a grandfather, or someone similar) to join the therapeutic "team." Aunts or Grandpas usually have enough emotional energy to cope with the problems that the traumatized child presents. Over the years I have successfully worked with children shifted from another country to live for a year in the United States with a relative (because they had been kidnapped), or youngsters brought into California from other parts of the United States for several weeks (kidnapping, stepparent abuse, destruction of a home), or adolescents separated from parents while attending a California high school or college. In each of these situations, one counsels the absent parents or primary caretaker by phone, in person, and (I suppose) by e-mail. I prefer the first 2, because they are immediate back-and-forth styles of communication, rather than letters. The idea is to let parents in on the treatment plan and then to get them to help augment its effectiveness.

Interventions with Schools, Hospitals, Churches, Coaches

Wherever traumatized children go, some help may be needed. One might consider the child's psychotherapist to be leader of a team of specialists that, in many instances, aids the youngster's recovery. If the child has an assigned attorney, the psychiatrist might convey the treatment plan to the lawyer. Symptoms should be explained to teachers, so they do not expel a traumatized child for sitting under a desk or needing extra times to go to the bathroom. The clinician must also hear about the child's symptoms outside of home so that, in psychotherapy sessions, they can be taken up and discussed, or played away. I mention "churches and coaches" because, depending on the child, these institutional personnel and policies may have a distinct bearing on the traumatized patient's well-being. What happens in a hospital after a trauma may further traumatize the child, or it can begin to assist the child on the road to recovery. The psychotherapist, of course, has ideas about this kind of intervention and should make sure to speak to the right individual to set the child in the proper direction.

CLINICAL CASE: INTERVENTIONS OUTSIDE THE HOME

A tall, 15-year-old girl of mixed American Indian and African American origins was sexually approached and frightened by her 19-year-old cousin. She fended him off several times, told her family about it, and experienced a breach in the family when her cousin's parents believed their son's story and disbelieved hers. The girl's parents brought her to me for trauma treatment; but it became clear after a couple of sessions that she felt satisfied she had handled the situation with her cousin. She knew about sex. She had been shocked at her cousin's advances but had let him know it was wrong. Though she had experienced a few bad dreams, she was not experiencing changes in personality or new directions in life. She was an ambitious athlete—actually a star at women's basketball—and she wanted to talk about that. She was attending a private high school that was almost entirely white. As a freshman, she had pushed her team to the county championship, yet she was granted no special notice, no awards. She was feeling more "traumatized" by basketball than by her cousin.

With her permission, I spoke to the coach. "Why," he wondered, "was she objecting? The rest of the team didn't like this girl—after all, she wasn't invited to their houses and they didn't speak with her much." I sensed that he and the team were prejudiced. I recommended a school with a greater mix of ethnicities. This girl needed a chance to be accepted by others. The family was able to find another private school for her, a good financial arrangement, and a basketball team (though considerably lower in ranking) to play on. She transferred schools. Her therapy ended. Four years later I followed-up by phone. The girl was now playing basketball at a top-level university. Yes, the more ethnically diverse school had helped her, and she had eventually helped her new school to a number-one position in their district. But no, the family breach had never been mended.

Mixing Modalities of Treatment

Cognitive-behavioral treatment (CBT) has been proven effective as a short-term therapy for childhood trauma.[43,44] The problem is, we don't know much about what happens long after these CBT treatments are over. They obviously help with contexts (the cognitive approach) and corrections (the behavioral approach). And they can be mixed in well with any other talking or playing modes of treatment. For instance, the psychodynamic therapist can easily ask a frightened youngster to try out a "homework assignment" as part of his treatment—say, to bring a ball to school for a few days and then later, to try playing 4-square at recess. One uses the principle of showing the child how to relax, and then asking the child to try actions from lower to higher on a chain of worrisome to downright frightening acts. CBT options can be mixed with playing a psychoanalytically derived "Dinosaur" game in the office, or with talking with a child about overexcited sexual feelings.

Medications may be used for traumatized children along with the psychotherapies. Some selective serotonin reuptake inhibitors were originally suggested for traumas, but then, many of them were deemed inadequately tested in young people. Clonidine, a central-acting agent that was considered useful for traumas in the 1980s, is not used very much today. The benzodiazepine tranquilizers can be used for a couple of weeks at a time, especially if a traumatic fear takes on a sudden resurgence. Benzodiazepines, however, are usually tapered off within weeks so that no habituation or cognitive blunting occurs. Antipsychotics have little utility in the treatment of trauma unless the young patient is suffering from posttraumatic delusions, hallucinations, or misperceptions ("psychotic" PTSD). If psychosis occurs, the antipsychotic medication need not stay in place long after the psychotic crisis is over. Finally, mood stabilizers (some of them well tested in children because they were used for years in treating seizure disorders) have not offered much to the treatment of trauma. Any of these medication options may be tried (with great caution, I might add), but the talk and play therapies appear to be the mainstays of childhood trauma therapy today.

TREATMENT THROUGH DEVELOPMENT

The meaning of a traumatic experience may change with each new developmental phase a child undergoes. At first, threats to attachment or autonomy may loom the largest. Later, injury or death may become key factors. Even later, the loss of a sense of identity may emerge as an issue. All along, life themes, established in the weeks and months following a trauma, are likely to stay in effect—now and then, gaining new variations based on the current stage of development.

In an ideal world, we would check traumatized kids at each new phase. (They go to their pediatricians for check-ups. Why not to us, as well?) At the present time, however, we must try to tell children and parents that trauma cannot be totally cured. It will flare up at times, sometimes because of a new external event and sometimes because of a new phase. We, or someone who does what we do, must be consulted early so that the whole disorder does not recur. A symptomatic recurrence can usually be dealt within a few weeks to months. New nightmares or a sudden reenactment does not necessarily mean a total return to "the drawing board." If childhood trauma was successfully treated once, the second treatment is usually shorter and easier.

The following are some examples of the kinds of developmental flares of which I write.

1. A girl, sexually abused orally in preschool by the provider's teenage son (proven), is treated psychodynamically in latency, and she does well. She phones her old therapist from college. She cannot stand intimate kissing. What should she do?
2. A boy, sexually abused by a male pedophile when he was 3 (proven), is treated as a preschooler and does well. At 13, a boy with whom he is staying overnight comes to his bed and tries to involve him in a sex act. The traumatized boy becomes concerned that he is "giving off gay vibes." He needs 3 months of psychodynamic therapy to fend off the resurgence of symptoms.
3. A 3-year-old who was kidnapped by her divorced father is returned to her mother after a year on the run. As a 4-year-old, she hates her mother for "giving me up." She is successfully treated but returns as an adult because she cannot let her mother retire. Her mom wants to move several miles away. "I depend on her being there for me," the child, now grown to womanhood, says. Once the doctor offers her a clear explanation of how close this comes to her old feelings as a 3-year-old child-napping victim, she accepts it, allowing her mom to fulfill her plans.

I end this review of trauma on an optimistic note. Psychodynamic psychotherapy works well for traumatized children.[30] In the meantime, before we obtain that long-term evidence-based proofs, consider treating traumas in childhood with abreaction, context, and correction. I have watched the results in the long run with many young patients, too many to exemplify on these pages. Each case teaches us something new. Each case offers a new problem to be solved. The joys of talking and playing with a child are inherent to every young patient we take on. So, difficult as it may feel—and as hard as it is to think of a child suffering—consider treating childhood trauma psychodynamically. It is a worthwhile pursuit, not just for the individual youngster, but for society as a whole. Some day in the future, a group of therapists may follow a large, same-age, similarly traumatized group into adulthood. Some "subjects" will receive psychodynamic psychotherapy and others, randomly selected, of course, will be given comparable current treatments. Over the long haul, psychodynamic psychotherapy will most likely demonstrate its efficacy. But it must be proven to do so.

REFERENCES

1. Freud A, Burlingham D. War and children. New York: Medical War Books; 1943. p. 68–9.
2. Terr L. Psychic trauma in children: observations following the Chowchilla school bus kidnapping. Am J Psychiatry 1981;138:14–9.
3. Terr L. Chowchilla revisited: the effects of psychic trauma four years after a schoolbus kidnapping. Am J Psychiatry 1983;140:1543–50.
4. Terr L. Life attitudes, dreams, and psychic trauma in a group of 'normal' children. J Am Acad Child Psychiatry 1983;22:221–30.
5. Pynoos R, Frederick C, Nader K, et al. Life threat and posttraumatic stress in school age children. Arch Gen Psychiatry 1987;44:1057–63.
6. Kinzie JD, Sack W, Angell R, et al. The psychiatric effects of massive trauma on Cambodian children. J Am Acad Child Adolesc Psychiatry 1986;25:370–85.
7. Kinzie JD, Sack W, Angell R, et al. A three-year follow-up of Cambodian young people traumatized as children. J Am Acad Child Adolesc Psychiatry 1989;28:501–4.
8. Sack WH, Clake G, Him C, et al. A 6-year follow-up study of Cambodian refugee adolescents traumatized as children. J Am Acad Child Adolesc Psychiatry 1993;32:431–7.
9. Eth S, Pynoos R. Interaction of trauma and grief in childhood. In: Eth S, Pynoos R, editors. Post-traumatic stress disorder in children. Washington (DC): Am Psychiatric Press; 1985. p. 169–86.
10. Hendriks JH, Black D, Kaplan T. When father kills mother. Guiding children through trauma and grief. London: Routledge; 1993.
11. Terr L. Childhood traumas: an outline and overview. Am J Psychiatry 1991;148:10–20.
12. Herman J. Trauma and recovery. New York: Basic Books; 1992.
13. Terr L. Too scared to cry. New York: Basic Books; 1992.
14. Terr L. The child as a witness. In: Schetky D, Benedek E, editors. Child psychiatry and the law. New York: Brunner Mazel; 1980. p. 207–21.
15. Terr L. 'Wild child': how three principles of healing organized 12 years of psychotherapy. J Am Acad Child Adolesc Psychiatry 2003;41:1401–9.
16. Levy D. Release therapy. Am J Orthop 1939;9:713–36.
17. Nader K, Schafe GE, LeDoux J. Fear memories require protein synthesis in the amygdala for reconsolidation after retrieval. Nature 2000;406:722–6.
18. Bogdan R, Williamson DE, Hariri AR. Mineralocorticoid receptor iso/val (rs 5522) genotype moderates the association between previous childhood emotional neglect and amygdala reactivity. Am J Psychiatry 2012;169:515–22.
19. Terr L. The use of context in the treatment of traumatized children. Psychoanal Study Child 2009;64:275–98.
20. Terr L. Children of Chowchilla: a study of psychic trauma. Psychoanal Study Child 1979;34:547–623.
21. Pynoos R. Traumatic stress and developmental psychopathology in children. In: Oldham JM, Riba MB, Tasman A, editors. Review of psychiatry 12. Washington (DC): American Psychiatric Press; 1993.
22. Terr L. Play therapy and psychic trauma: a preliminary report. In: Schaefer C, O'Conner K, editors. Handbook of play therapy. New York: John Wiley & Sons; 1983. p. 308–19.
23. Furman E. Filial therapy. In: Noshpitz J, editor. Basic handbook of child psychiatry, vol. 3. New York: Basic Books; 1979. p. 149–58.

24. Landreth GL, Bratton SC. Child parent relationship therapy (CPRT). New York: Routledge; 2006.
25. Loftus EF. Desperately seeking memories of the first few years of childhood: the reality of early memories. J Exp Psychol Gen 1993;122:274–7.
26. Saywitz KJ, Goodman GS, Nicholas E, et al. Children's memories of physical examinations involving genital touch. J Consult Clin Psychol 1991;59:682–91.
27. Pynoos R, Nader K. Children's memory and proximity to violence. J Am Acad Child Adolesc Psychiatry 1989;28:236–41.
28. Terr L. What happens to early memories of trauma? J Am Acad Child Adolesc Psychiatry 1988;27:96–104.
29. Yates A, Terr L. Anatomically correct dolls: should they be used as the basis for expert testimony? J Am Acad Child Adolesc Psychiatry 1988;27:254–7, 387–8.
30. Terr L. Magical moments of change. New York: Norton; 2008.
31. Brody M. Holy franchise! Batman and trauma. In: Rubin L, editor. Using superheroes in counseling and play therapy. New York: Springer; 2007. p. 105–20.
32. Gardner R. Therapeutic communication with children: the mutual story telling technique. New York: Science House; 1971.
33. Emde R, Wolf D, Oppenheim D. Revealing the inner worlds of young children. New York: Oxford; 2003.
34. Terr L. "Forbidden games": post-traumatic child's play. J Am Acad Child Psychiatry 1981;20:741–60.
35. Gaensbauer TJ. Traumatized young children: assessment and treatment process. In: Osofsky JD, editor. Young children and trauma: intervention and treatment. New York: Guilford; 2004. p. 194–215.
36. Chethik M. Techniques of child therapy—psychodynamic strategies. 2nd edition. New York: Guilford; 2000.
37. Carey L. Sandplay therapy with children and families. Northvale (NJ): Aronson; 1999.
38. Knell SM. Cognitive behavioral play therapy. In: Shaefer C, editor. Foundations of play therapy. Hoboken, NJ: Wiley; 2003. p. 175–91.
39. Benham AL, Slotnick CF. Play therapy: integrating clinical and developmental perspectives. In: Luby JL, editor. Handbook of infant mental health. New York: Guilford; 2006. p. 331–69.
40. Webb NB, editor. Play therapy with children in crisis. 3rd edition. New York: Guilford; 2007.
41. Greenspan SI. Developmentally based psychotherapy. Madison (CT): International University Press; 1997.
42. Fraiberg S. Ghosts in the nursery. In: Fraiberg L, editor. Selected writings of Selma Fraiberg. Columbus (OH): Ohio State University Press; 1987. p. 100–36.
43. Cohen JA, Mannarino AP, Deblinger S. Treating trauma and traumatic grief in children and adolescents. New York: Guilford; 2006.
44. Knell SM. Cognitive behavioral play therapy. Northvale (NJ): Jason Aronson; 1993.

Psychodynamic Psychotherapy as Treatment for Depression in Adolescence

Nick Midgley, MSc, PsychD*, Simon Cregeen, MPsychPsych, Carol Hughes, BA (Psych), Margaret Rustin, BA Hons

KEYWORDS

• Depression • Adolescence • Psychotherapy • Psychoanalytic • Psychodynamic • IMPACT Study

KEY POINTS

- Encouraging indications from research studies are that short-term psychodynamic psychotherapy (STPP) may be effective for the treatment of internalizing disorders and, in particular, child and adolescent depression.
- Psychodynamic therapy may be the treatment of choice for depressed teenagers with complex, chronic difficulties and comorbidities, whereby the emphasis is on supporting the developmental process more broadly rather than focusing exclusively on a reduction of symptoms.
- Attentiveness to unconscious phenomena is specific to psychodynamic psychotherapy, is related to the theoretical importance attributed to these deep layers of the mind, and is closely linked to the techniques used by the therapist.
- Both therapist and young person need to be wary of the omnipotent fantasy of the "total cure" and be able to work toward a more realistic sense of a "good enough" ending.

Josie had just turned 15 when she began her psychotherapy. She was brought to her first appointment by her father and sister, who stayed in the room with Josie throughout the meeting. Once seated Josie was almost silent, except for saying quietly "I don't know how I got to be here." Later in the session, once her family had told the story of how Josie had become depressed and taken an overdose, the therapist was able to draw her out on this. Josie said "I was a little girl and then one day I was a teenager. I don't know how I got to be here. It's like I'm in a faraway country. I am lost. I don't know where to go or what to do."

INTRODUCTION: DEPRESSION IN ADOLESCENCE

According to a report funded by the World Bank and the World Health Organization,[1] depression is the leading cause of disability in the world, with over half of mental

Anna Freud Centre, 21 Maresfield Gardens, London NW3 2HX, UK
* Corresponding author.
E-mail address: nickmidgley@btconnect.com

Child Adolesc Psychiatric Clin N Am 22 (2013) 67–82
http://dx.doi.org/10.1016/j.chc.2012.08.004 **childpsych.theclinics.com**
1056-4993/13/$ – see front matter

Key Abbreviations: Adolescent Depression	
CBT	Cognitive-behavioral therapy
IMPACT	Improving Mood with Psychoanalytic and Cognitive-Behavioural Therapy study
LTPP	Long-term psychodynamic psychotherapy
NICE	National Institute for Health and Clinical Excellence
STPP	Short-term psychodynamic psychotherapy

health costs in Europe each year going toward the treatment of people suffering from anxiety and depression. Among those suffering from clinical depression, more than 60% report that they first suffered from depression during their teenage years. The outcomes for those who become depressed as adolescents are not encouraging, with a high risk of a range of illnesses in later life, including increased rates of self harm, suicide, and other mental and physical health problems, compared with other adolescents.[2,3] It is therefore vital that effective interventions are developed that not only offer support when young people first experience depression but also help to promote the kind of resilience that will prevent long-term mental health problems from developing. Treatments such as cognitive-behavioral therapy (CBT) have been shown to be effective, at least in the short term, for those with mild to moderate depression. But the evidence for the long-term effectiveness of CBT, especially for more severe depression, is mixed.[4] In the authors' view psychodynamic psychotherapy, when seen as part of a multidisciplinary intervention, has a significant contribution to make as a treatment option for young people with depression.

PSYCHODYNAMIC PSYCHOTHERAPY AS A TREATMENT OPTION FOR DEPRESSION IN ADOLESCENCE

Compared with some other therapies, psychodynamic treatment has lagged in developing a robust evidence base, but the pace of research is now accelerating.[a] In a recent systematic review of the evidence base, Midgley and Kennedy[5] identified 35 distinct research studies, including 9 randomized controlled trials, which evaluated the effectiveness or efficacy of psychodynamic work with children and young people. The review suggested that there is a small, but growing, body of evidence in support of the effectiveness of child and adolescent psychodynamic psychotherapy, with especially encouraging indications that short-term psychodynamic psychotherapy (STPP) may be effective for the treatment of internalizing disorders[6,7] and, in particular, child and adolescent depression.[8–10] The study by Trowell and colleagues[10,11] is important because it demonstrated that although young people engaged in short-term psychodynamic psychotherapy showed slower initial rates of improvement than those receiving systemic family therapy, by the end of treatment both therapies were effective. Moreover, the gains made by those young people receiving psychodynamic therapy were maintained and even increased during a 1-year follow-up period.

The evidence for both long-term psychodynamic psychotherapy and STPP in the treatment of adults is more substantial, with several studies focusing on the psychodynamic treatment of depression.[12–15] Clinical practice guidelines for the treatment of depression in adults identified STPP as demonstrating effectiveness

[a] The term "psychodynamic psychotherapy" is used here as a generic term for a range of treatments informed by psychoanalytic principles. In the United Kingdom, child and adolescent psychotherapists are seen as providing psychoanalytic therapy; they are trained to provide both intensive psychoanalytic therapy and a range of other work, including assessment, brief interventions, work with parents, supervision, and consultation to other professionals.

comparable with that of other psychological therapies and medication.[16] There are some indications that for major depression, combined treatment (psychodynamic and medication) is more effective than either one alone.[17] Moreover, a recent meta-analysis suggested that there was clear evidence for effectiveness, superiority over controls, and comparability with other therapies in follow-up, but marginal inferiority in some measures in immediate follow-up.[18] The investigators concluded that more and higher-quality studies of STPP were needed if it is to meet criteria for an empirically supported treatment; this holds equally true for STPP with both adults and children.

Improving Mood with Psychoanalytic and Cognitive-Behavioural Therapy Study

As part of developing such an evidence base, the authors of this article are members of the STPP steering group for a large-scale clinical trial currently under way in the United Kingdom, the Improving Mood with Psychoanalytic and Cognitive-Behavioural Therapy Study (IMPACT) (Midgley N, Cregeen S, Hughes C, et al. Short-term psychoanalytic psychotherapy (STPP) for adolescents with moderate to severe depression. A treatment manual. 2010. Version 1. Submitted for publication).[4] This randomized controlled trial aims to investigate the role of psychological therapies in reducing relapse for adolescents with moderate to severe depression. The findings of this study, the largest clinical trial to examine psychodynamic work with young people ever performed, are likely to go a long way toward establishing more confidently whether short-term psychodynamic therapy can be considered an evidence-based treatment for adolescent depression. In the meantime, this article sets out a psychodynamic approach to both understanding and treating adolescent depression. This approach is based largely on the manual for STPP for adolescents (11–17 years old) with moderate to severe depression, developed for the IMPACT study (Midgley N, Cregeen S, Hughes C, et al. Short-term psychoanalytic psychotherapy (STPP) for adolescents with moderate to severe depression. A treatment manual. 2010. Version 1. Submitted for publication). Although this article makes reference to longer-term psychodynamic treatments, the 28-session model (plus 7 sessions of parent/carer work) used in the IMPACT study informs the psychodynamic approach presented here.

A PSYCHOANALYTIC UNDERSTANDING OF THE DEVELOPMENT OF DEPRESSION IN ADOLESCENCE

Josie lives with her birth parents, Mr and Mrs B, and her younger brother Kenny (5 years old). Josie has an older sister Rebecca (19) who recently became engaged and moved in with her fiancé. Mrs B has long-standing mental health difficulties which have affected her capacity to care for her children. Rebecca had been a major caregiver for her younger siblings, a role that Josie was expected to take on for her brother, Kenny, when her older sister started work and became engaged. Josie has a difficult relationship with her mother, by whom she is both verbally and emotionally attacked with threats and criticism.

Josie is an intelligent young woman, who was an academic high achiever. It seemed that her sister's engagement precipitated the depressive breakdown. Until that point Rebecca had been a protective factor in Josie's life. Alongside this, the developmental challenges of the move into puberty and adolescence proved too much for Josie. She attempted to deal with these challenges through a premature (asexual) romantic relationship with a boy from school, which contained within it a fantasy of oneness (denying the need to develop her own separate identity). With the loss of this relationship (and the defensive fantasy) as well as the "loss" of her sister, Josie collapsed into depression, feeling hopeless, defeated, and unable to face the future. It was at this point that she tried to take her own life.

TWO PSYCHOANALYTIC FORMULATIONS OF DEPRESSION

Rooted in the work of Freud,[19] Abraham,[20] and Klein,[21] early psychoanalysts offered an understanding of depression as related to loss, guilt and a sense of responsibility for having attacked and damaged the ambivalently loved or lost object. "Object" is a term in psychoanalysis that refers both to significant external figures (particularly parental), and to internal representations of those figures. These internal representations are developed on the basis of lived experiences (especially early in life) with carers and parents, and through the individual's own emotional attitude toward, and toleration of, such lived experiences. Internal objects both reflect directly the reality of external figures and are significantly shaped by the individual's own projective and introjective processes. The world of internal objects is a dynamic conception and, hence, forever in movement and subject to change. The outcome of such guilt was understood to be a sense of the self as worthless, bad, and potentially destructive, and the typical depressive symptoms, such as self-criticism and the wish to die, were understood as the behavioral manifestation of these underlying dynamics.

Since the 1970s there has been an increasing interest among psychoanalysts in issues related to narcissistic vulnerability and "narcissistic depression."[22] Kernberg,[23] for example, writes of a certain type of depression "which has more of the quality of impotent rage, or of helplessness-hopelessness in connection with the breakdown of an idealized self-concept." A chronic sense of emptiness, often a result of failures in empathic parenting, was described by Kohut[24] as the core depressive feature in some narcissistic patients. Alongside the emphasis on guilt owing to a sense of having damaged the object, in this type of depression, according to Kohut, there is a greater focus on the subject's own sense of narcissistic fragility, with subsequent feelings of shame and humiliation. The empirical research literature provides some support for the idea that these 2 formulations capture different subtypes of depression, at least for adults, each one describing a group of depressed individuals with differing presentations and differing vulnerabilities, and with potentially differing responses to therapy.[25]

Depression Formulated as a Developmental Crisis

For young people, any understanding of depressive dynamics has to be put in the context of normal developmental processes.[26] Psychoanalysts writing about adolescence have stressed its importance as the time during which the young person consolidates his or her own independent identity. Whereas investigators such as Erikson[27] and Blos[28] have emphasized the achievement of autonomy, others such as the Laufers[29] have focused on the impact of developing a sexual body. The emotional-developmental tasks of adolescence inevitably involve the reemergence of Oedipal anxieties, feelings, and conflicts that were first met and wrestled with in toddlerhood.[21] For many adolescents the active mobilization of Oedipal dynamics can be a startling and confusing experience. Adolescence presents an opportunity to rework Oedipal matters (now in the context of a sexually maturing body) and eventually establish a secure young adult sexual and relational identity. However, the task can also be felt to be too much—even threatening—and lead to developmental retreat, a turning away, or manic and promiscuous activity.[30] Vulnerable youngsters with limited, inflexible, or primitive defenses and an insecurely established ego (sense of self) often find adolescent developmental tasks overwhelming. In this sense, adolescent depression can be viewed as a developmental crisis. In turn, the hopeless withdrawal that is characteristic of depression means that the young person cannot engage in the activities and relationships of his or her peers, so that a vicious circle may be set in motion.

The challenges of adolescence are more pronounced for those young people who have had significant histories of difficulties in the parent-infant or early parent-child relationships.[31] It seems that if these difficulties involved closeness or enmeshment, then youngsters may demonstrate considerable difficulties in individuating in adolescence. By contrast, if the early relationships were marked by distance, quite often adolescents seem to hurtle into adolescent relationships, sometimes into promiscuous sexuality and risk-taking behavior such as drug or alcohol abuse (Hughes and colleagues, unpublished data, 2012). These young people may be seeking emotional closeness, not necessarily sexual gratification, although the two are often conflated in a confused way. The expectations of these relationships are unrealistic, with a wish for "oneness" and a fantasy of all emotional needs being met. Such expectations are fragile and often result in relationship breakdown, which triggers further loss and a sense of abandonment and evokes depressive symptoms. In Josie's case, at the age of 14 she developed an intense relationship with a boy who lived nearby, in which the two of them "felt like we were one person, we always knew what the other one was thinking." The breakup of this relationship clearly precipitated her depression, although it was only with a second loss (when her sister left the family home) that Josie broke down more overtly. In the authors' clinical experience, many adolescent suicide attempts are in the context of such losses. For such young people, it may be that the move into an adolescent state of mind is experienced as the total loss of a psychic "home." For others, it may lead to a despairing realization of the fragility of their link with good and sustaining internal and external objects.

Such a fragile sense of a "core self" has been noted as a common feature of depressed adolescents in the clinical literature.[32] Rhode[33] speaks of depressed children and adolescents with profound annihilation anxieties, who in treatment expressed the belief that they were living in a "black hole": that they did not feel they existed, or had the right to exist.[33] For example, once Josie's mood lifted she described how being depressed had felt as if she were liquid: "I felt sorta like water, liquid, just draining away. In fact, I wanted to soak away, just not to be anymore. Now I am not depressed I feel kind of solid. The wind can blow, I am solid—I am here."

Depression Formulated as "Conflicted Anger"

Clinical experience suggests that many depressed youngsters also present with what Busch and colleagues[34] have called conflicted anger. Because such anger is felt to be unacceptable, it may be split off and denied and/or consequently break through in aggressive outbursts, which can leave them and their families distressed. Josie, for example, would on rare occasions have sudden outbursts of anger, during which she would smash some of her favorite possessions in her room, in a way that left her parents feeling that this behavior had "appeared out of nowhere." Afterward she would be left feeling guilty and confused, bereft at having damaged objects that she cared about and unable to explain why she had been so angry.

Integrated aggression, in the form of appropriate assertiveness and testing out of intellectual strength and personal passions in the service of the development of the personality, is rare among depressed teenagers. For some, the parent is perceived as being too fragile to survive and so is protected by an internalization of the anger, turning it onto the adolescent self. This process can take the form of self hatred and reproach as well as physical attacks of the self through cutting or self harm. Some depressed youngsters feel, in an unrealistic, omnipotent way, that their anger and aggression is too dangerous and that is has somehow caused their parents' mental illness or fragility. When this is the case it has important implications for treatment, as at some stage it is likely that this disavowed anger and aggression is likely to reappear in the treatment, focused on the relationship with the therapist (the transference). When it does so, there is a high risk of treatment breakdown or of acting out behavior, unless the anger can be addressed directly and the young person made to feel safe enough to explore in the context of a containing relationship with the therapist. As Josie put it quite late on in her therapy (after several difficult sessions, during which she had been very challenging to her therapist): "at times I really hated you; but I always knew that you were on my side."

INDICATIONS FOR REFERRAL FOR PSYCHODYNAMIC PSYCHOTHERAPY FOR ADOLESCENT DEPRESSION

The child psychiatrist who met Josie and her parents immediately after she had taken an overdose concluded that Josie was not at immediate risk of further self harm, but he did think that Josie needed further help. He discussed medication but, based on his assessment, the psychiatrist considered that they should "watch and wait" before deciding whether to go ahead with a course of fluoxetine. Instead he suggested that Josie might be helped by CBT. However, Josie's parents said to the psychiatrist that Josie had already been offered CBT at school a few months earlier, and hadn't been able to manage the cognitive tasks that were set for her. Josie agreed that she didn't want to try this again. In speaking to Josie alone, the psychiatrist wondered whether she might benefit from a less structured setting than CBT, where she could use her interest in drawing to express what she was feeling. He suggested that Josie meet with a child and adolescent psychotherapist in the team instead, and Josie agreed to this. Soon after, an assessment for psychodynamic therapy was begun.

In the United Kingdom, the present guidance provided by the National Institute for Health and Clinical Excellence suggests a stepped-care approach to the treatment of child and adolescent depression, with time-limited psychodynamic psychotherapy (up to 30 sessions) considered only for those patients not responsive to standard psychoeducational support and family work, or to brief cognitive-behavioral input.[35] This guidance also suggests that some types of antidepressant medication should be considered alongside psychotherapy, especially for more severe depression if clinically appropriate. The guidance also stresses that the "best available evidence" should be considered alongside the professional judgment of the clinician, taking into account the preferences of the service user. So in Josie's case, a referral to psychodynamic therapy took place directly following her initial assessment with a child psychiatrist.

There is not yet enough empirical research to say with confidence which depressed young people are most likely to benefit from psychodynamic interventions, although the IMPACT study[4] described earlier should provide some data on this matter. However, clinical experience suggests that psychodynamic therapy is often the treatment of choice for depressed teenagers with complex, chronic difficulties and comorbidities, whereby the emphasis may be on supporting the developmental process more broadly rather than focusing exclusively on a reduction of symptoms.[36]

Even in time-limited (and focused) treatment, psychodynamic psychotherapists address the whole personality of the patient and the whole nexus of object relationships, both internalized and current. Using the terms of Luyten and Blatt,[37] the treatment is person-centered, not disorder-centered. As most depressed young people referred to child and adolescent mental health services have a range of other difficulties and diagnoses (eg, anxiety, compromised attachment, obsessional symptoms, or conduct disorders), the wide perspective of psychodynamic therapy addresses both the depressive phenomena and other significant personality factors or disorders that are likely to be interacting with the depression. The treatment may be particularly suitable when there has been a long history of difficulties and where there are intergenerational continuities (eg, a history of parental depression) and entanglements. Dependence on a highly rigid defensive system would be a contraindication for treatment. Psychodynamic therapy is also not recommended when there are child protection issues that have not yet been adequately addressed.

DEVELOPING A PSYCHOANALYTIC FORMULATION TO GUIDE TREATMENT

The initial meetings between Josie and her psychotherapist established that she was a bright, high-achieving girl, whose previously "warm" personality had changed about 6 months before her referral. At the time of the referral, Josie met the Diagnostic and Statistical Manual of Mental Disorders (DSM) diagnostic criteria for Major Depression (moderate). Although she was no longer actively suicidal at the time of the therapy assessment, she continued to be depressed, had thoughts about self harm, and was not attending school. She was said by her parents to have gone from being a girl with a full life with plans for her future to lying on her bed, tearful and apathetic.

As well as assessing her symptoms, the therapist was interested to get a picture of Josie's "internal world" and to develop some initial hypotheses about what had gone wrong with Josie's development. During one of the initial meetings, Josie described throwing herself into an intense asexual romantic relationship with a boy of her age. "We were like one person. We didn't even need to say anything—we just knew what we each felt or thought." When this relationship broke down she tipped into severe depression and tried to take her life through an overdose. The therapist understood this as a collapse in the face of the unbearable loss she experienced as she faced separation and individuation. Paradoxically she tried to "find herself" through psychic merger with this boy, and experienced the subsequent loss as a loss of her own sense of self. Josie tried to defend herself against unwanted feelings in several ways. She located the need for care in her brother (compulsive caregiving); she avoided family tensions by withdrawing and thereby disowning her own anger (until it occasionally broke out in unmanageable ways); and finally, all capacity for separation and having one's own voice was located in other people. This left her emptied of parts of herself and ego capacities, and she collapsed emotionally. She retreated from a seemingly threatening external world and stopped going to school. As such a range of psychosomatic illnesses provided Josie with a form of escapism, as she could take to her bed and be left "undisturbed" by the rest of the family. It seemed that Josie was afraid that her aggression would damage an already fragile object (a parent with a mental illness), and so she turned it on herself.

A "case formulation", such as the (abbreviated) one given here, is an important element in framing psychoanalytic work, especially short-term or time-limited psychotherapy. In addition to data gathered from the initial meetings with the young person, this assessment draws on family information derived from the parent worker, any initial assessment meetings with the other child and adolescent mental health service clinicians, plus demographic and psychiatric data made available to the clinician from formal assessments that may be used. As well as the standard information about the referral, developmental history, and a statement regarding protective and risk factors, a psychodynamic formulation would include a statement outlining the therapist's initial hypotheses about central psychodynamic features and how they maintain the young person's depression and/or make the young person vulnerable to depressive moods, within a dynamic developmental context. Busch and colleagues[34] present an integrated psychodynamic formulation for depression in adults that is based around an assessment of 5 key areas, which the authors have found helpful. This formulation is presented in **Box 1** (with some adaptations to take into account the differences between adults and adolescents).

Without focusing treatment too narrowly on any one particular element of the presenting problems, a preliminary formulation helps to define the field of attention for the therapeutic work by concentrating on underlying psychodynamic issues. This approach may be especially important in STPP, where it is essential that treatment focuses on identified dynamics, defenses, and issues that have been spoken about in a meaningful way with the adolescent.[38]

THE AIMS OF PSYCHODYNAMIC TREATMENT FOR DEPRESSED ADOLESCENTS

At first Josie couldn't manage without her father or a friend in the therapy room, feeling she didn't know what she felt or how to describe what was happening to her. Only later in the therapy did she feel able to come into the room on her own. Over time she and her therapist came to understand how the onset of adolescence took her unawares, despite her physical maturation. She was not emotionally ready to be a teenager. Now that she was in therapy, she spoke of wanting to find "her old self" again, and to discover ways that would help her cope if she ever felt so depressed that she wanted to die again. She began to see that her depression was a "marker" that things weren't right in how she felt about herself as a person, and she wanted to try and change that "before it is too late."

Especially when working with time-limited psychodynamic psychotherapy, the clinician needs to bear in mind Winnicott's[39] point, that one may not be asking "how much

Box 1
Five elements commonly found in a psychodynamic formulation of depression

1. Narcissistic vulnerability; that is, an insecure sense of a separate self and a heightened sensitivity to perceived or actual losses and rejections leading to a lowering of self esteem, which in turn triggers depressive affects, existential angst, and rage in response to narcissistic injury.
2. Conflicted anger; that is, anger, blame, and envy directed toward others leads to disruptions in interpersonal relationships, confusion over responsibility and to self-directed anger and subsequent depressive affects.
3. Severe superego, experience of guilt and shame; that is, feelings and wishes seen as bad and/or wrong, with doubt about whether the young person's love outweighs aggression, leads to negative self-perceptions and self-criticism, and in some cases confusion between reality and fantasy.
4. Idealized and devalued expectations of self/others; that is, high self-expectations and/or idealization of others, often switching to sudden de-idealization and devaluation, may lead to disappointment, anger at self and others, and subsequent lowering of self esteem.
5. Characteristic means of defending against painful affects; that is, use of defenses typical to depression such as denial, projection, passive aggression, and reaction formations leading to increased depression because either the world is seen as hostile or the self is attacked. Splitting, as a characteristic defense against aggression, blocks assertive/aggressive efforts from integration in the service of personality development.

Data from Busch F, Rudden M, Shapiro T, editors. Psychodynamic treatment of depression. Washington, DC: American Psychiatric Publishing; 2004.

can one do?", but rather "what is the least that needs to be done?" Both therapist and young person need to be wary of the omnipotent fantasy of the "total cure," and be able to work toward a more realistic sense of a "good enough" ending.[40]

When the main features of the central depression dynamic are addressed successfully, outcomes of the treatment may include the following (see Busch and colleagues[34]):

- The young person can manage depressive feelings and aggression better
- The young person is less prone to guilt and self devaluation
- The young person can make more realistic assessments of his or her own behavior and motivation, and that of others
- The young person has a better developed sense of agency
- The young person has a better capacity to be thoughtful rather than to "act out"
- The young person has a more realistic view of what he or she is responsible for, and of the difference between fantasy and reality
- The young person is less vulnerable to depression in the face of loss, disappointment, and criticism

In Josie's case, the therapist and Josie's family were able to agree that they hoped to see her not only wanting to live and better able to attend school, but to recognize that this would depend on her being able to manage depressive feelings better and building up a greater resilience. The therapist had a hypothesis that helping Josie to become more aware of her aggressive feelings would be an important focus, but at the time of starting therapy this was not explicitly shared by the therapist, as it seemed important to allow Josie to begin treatment and find things out for herself.

THE TECHNIQUE OF PSYCHODYNAMIC PSYCHOTHERAPY WITH DEPRESSED YOUNG PEOPLE

Much of Josie's early therapy was conducted in silence. She chose to draw, her drawings being dark and forbidding. There were disturbing scenes of death: decaying cadavers, bloody skulls transfixed by daggers, and wounded bodies with bleeding gashes. Josie seemed absorbed in these images as well as in the process of image making. She seemed to "attack" the paper with pencil and black pens. Her therapist found herself watching and thinking intently, mirroring the intensity of Josie's preoccupation.

The ending of sessions was difficult. Josie found it hard to leave, often weeping, saying she couldn't face going. The therapist found herself terribly afraid that Josie would die before they met again, so she found herself extending the length of sessions—but they were never long enough. With the help of supervision, the therapist realized that Josie was not actively suicidal, but that she was allowing the therapist to get a sense of what Bion called a "nameless dread"[41] that Josie, herself, was protecting against through "projective identification."[41–43] Once the therapist was aware of this it was possible to manage her own anxiety, help Josie to feel that her anxieties could be thought about, and so end the sessions on time rather than "acting out in the countertransference" by prolonging the sessions.[44,45] (Supervision within psychodynamic psychotherapy has a vital role to play, dealing as we are, with unconscious processes, transference and countertransference phenomena. Consequently, within the IMPACT study STPP psychotherapists are required to attend regular supervision. The authors have manualized the process of psychotherapy supervision as a subsection of the STPP IMPACT manual. [Midgley N, Cregeen S, Hughes C, et al. Short-term psychoanalytic psychotherapy (STPP) for adolescents with moderate to severe depression. A treatment manual. 2010. Version 1. Submitted for publication.])

Josie's transference feelings toward her therapist were especially difficult in sessions before a break or in the whole period leading up to the end of therapy. By working through the ups and downs of her relationship with her therapist, Josie became better able to manage her anxieties about separation. As treatment entered the "middle phase," the therapist noticed a shift both in Josie and in her own countertransference. Although the actions seemed the same, the emotional tone changed from terror to anger. The therapist judged that Josie's internal object was now more robust and could withstand Josie's anger. She drew the rage into the transference by helping Josie to voice the rarely expressed feelings of anger and irritation toward her therapist. In doing so the therapist was allowing Josie an experience of being angry with the therapist and the therapist surviving. The therapist did not retaliate but remained a thinking person who could validate, process, and understand Josie's feelings. At this point Josie herself suddenly demanded to return to school, as if she had re-discovered a sense of assertion, a positive aggression, which allowed her to feel more potent and less terrified of the consequences of her anger. "I want to get on with my life," she told her therapist, "not be at the beck and call of my family."

Establishing a Psychodynamic Frame for the Therapy

The techniques of psychodynamic psychotherapy are primarily based on close and detailed observation of the relationship the young person makes with the therapist, and the theoretical assumption that the young person's free play, drawings, and conversation can be seen as equivalent to "free association." A suitable consulting room is required. Sessions take place in this same room and at the same time each week for ongoing therapy. The therapist introduces the context to the young person as one for understanding feelings and difficulties in his or her life. Undirected play, art activities, and talking are the fundamental sources of the relevant "clinical facts."[46]

The therapist's stance is nonjudgmental and enquiring, and conveys the value of words. The aim is to put into words the therapist's understanding of what the young person communicates through play, behavior, and verbal expression; this will include conscious and unconscious thoughts and feelings. Ritvo[36] proposes that the techniques used in psychodynamic treatment lie on a continuum, "from those that are most supportive of the patient's strengths and current adaptations to those which lead to expression of deeper feelings and bring the patient's inner conflicts and issues into the discussion."[36(p15)] In her actions and words, the therapist attempts to convey openness to all forms of psychic experience (current preoccupations, memories, daydreams, fantasies, and dreams) but will be attuned specifically to evidence of unconscious fantasies that underlie the young person's relationship to self and others. This attentiveness to unconscious phenomena is specific to psychodynamic psychotherapy, is related to the theoretical importance attributed to these deep layers of the mind, and is closely linked to the techniques used by the therapist.

These principles underlie the focus on the transference relationship made to the therapist, that is, the relationship made not in response to "real" aspects of the therapist's person and behavior, but arising from characteristics of the figures of the child or young person's internal world. These aspects are then believed to be present in the therapist, as a consequence of the externalization of the young person's picture of the world. Systematic observation of these transference elements allows for clarification of the young person's fundamental assumptions about the external world. The anxieties that underlie these beliefs can be analyzed and discussed, thus enabling the young person to begin to differentiate psychic from external reality. As a result, the adolescent may become more able to test out reality, and establish a fruitful relationship with it. Such an idea bears some similarity to Bowlby's concept of "internal working models" of attachment,[47–49] based on early experiences with our primary caregivers, but which may prove maladaptive in a new environment. Being able to develop new representations and expectations of others is an important part of therapeutic change, but is a slow process, requiring testing and retesting in the "here and now" of the therapeutic relationship.

Working with the Transference and the Countertransference

A central source of information to the therapist in expanding his or her understanding are the emotional responses evoked in him or her by the young person. These responses are broadly referred to as countertransference phenomena.[47] Such phenomena can include personal factors that intrude and distort the therapist's capacity for objective understanding, but also many responses arising from primitive nonverbal forms of communication, projective identifications, which the therapist becomes aware of. These are similar to the ways in which infants can communicate with their caretakers before the development of language, and depend on emotional availability and space for "reverie" in the therapist.[41] These primitive modes of relationship can be used to control anxiety by ridding oneself of it and pushing it outside rather than using it for communicative purposes. The distinction between benign (communicative) and malign (destructive, eg, to cause confusion) forms of projection is vital in clinical work. At times, for example, the anxiety that Josie's therapist felt about her safety was an important way that she could become alert to fragile states of mind that Josie herself was denying. At other times, in a more destructive way, the therapist would be left feeling so stupid and worthless at the end of a meeting with Josie that she just "couldn't think," and in those cases supervision became vital in helping her to see what painful feelings Josie herself was defending herself against by means of such malign projections.

With all adolescents, most particularly those with environmentally compromised early experiences, there is a need for the therapist to be in a state of mind characterized by availability to the reception of projected contents (anxieties, affects, uncertainties) of the adolescent's mind. These contents are often of a primitive nature and are not always known to the adolescents themselves. The patient's experience of the therapist receiving, holding in mind, and thinking about this projected material is a central feature of the work. Bion[50] describes how the placement and residence of toxic, primitive states of mind in the therapist's mind can lead to their detoxification. Previously unthinkable anxieties and emotions can then become thinkable, and in due course "returned" to the patient. Patients thereby gain ownership of a previously disowned part of themselves, and are strengthened by identification with an object experienced in this way.

PSYCHODYNAMIC TREATMENT IN A MULTIMODAL TREATMENT PLAN

Josie's parents (Michelle and David) were offered a space to meet a "parent worker" separately from Josie's meetings with her therapist. Concerns about the emotional environment in the family and Michelle's own mental health, and consequent multiagency involvement, helped gather and heighten the parents' awareness of the imperative for them to engage in some work themselves. Michelle's initial wariness, fear, and unfamiliarity with emotions being "thinkable about" and put into words, soon gave way to some relief that this was possible, given the right relational conditions. This process was an extremely painful one, as it led to realizations of how, as a parent to Josie, she had dealt with her own childhood experiences of being subject to parental cruelty and abandonment by behaving in the same way toward her daughter. Through this, Josie had been left as the one to feel helpless, criticized, despairing, and emotionally unplaced.

David attended the parent work sessions less frequently to begin with, but thanks to the clinician's persistence, David and Michelle eventually began attending parent work sessions together. The clinician was able to begin to help them think, as a parental couple, about Josie, and to see how David's fear of his own aggression was part of the reason why he was unable to protect his children adequately against Michelle's explosive rages. This joint work was an opportunity to strengthen the positive aspects of their relationship. The parents were also helped to see how their own painful, early experiences had made it more difficult for them to bring Josie up without exposing her to similar experiences, despite their active wish to avoid this. Although painful for them, this awareness was an important step in allowing the parents to do things differently, in the way they had always hoped.

Importance of a Multidisciplinary Team

Psychodynamic treatment with severely depressed adolescents needs to be considered in relation to the various contexts of the young people's lives, and within a multidisciplinary team framework. This notion reflects the fact that adolescent depression is in most cases multiply determined,[51] and as such needs to be treated in an integrated way. We need no longer see genetics and environmental factors, physiology, and psychology as "either/or," but can see the "both/and" in the complex interplay of these factors. Goodyer,[52] for example, points to the complexity of brain, hormonal, and family factors, and life events, which interact in adolescent depression. The psychotherapist and/or parent worker requires alertness to the need, at times, for active communication and liaison with other significant individuals and agencies in the adolescent's life. This liaison may include external agencies such as school/college, youth and social services, and mental health colleagues, most particularly child and adolescent psychiatrists (if the therapist is not one him or herself), especially when there are issues about risk and a possible need for medication or hospitalization.

Parent Work

Therapeutic work with parents or carers offered concurrently and in parallel with an adolescent's psychodynamic psychotherapy (by different clinicians) is a well-established practice in the work of most psychodynamic child and adolescent therapists in the United Kingdom,[53–55] and there is some evidence that psychodynamic therapy is more effective when offered alongside parent work.[5] In relation to their son's or daughter's depressive difficulties, parents may be struggling in several ways: for instance, under the pressures of living with them ("I can't bear it"), under the pressure of parental guilt ("is this because of me?") or fear ("what might they do?"), or under the pressure of identification ("I was like this at their age" or "I am still like this at 40") and despair ("nothing has helped"). In addition to engaging the parents in the treatment process, the therapeutic relationship with the parent worker aims to help contain parental anxieties, and gives space to think about their relationship to their son or daughter. An associated task is to help the parents create space in their minds to re-imagine their child in fresh and previously unknown ways, to foster their capacity for reflective functioning.[56]

As a model of change, if parental anxieties are emotionally contained, they are better placed to think about their experience as a parent, which includes emotions and anxieties aroused within them by their depressed son or daughter. Parent work can enable the parents to think anew, or more freely, about adolescent development and how to support this. Being less anxiously invaded by the adolescent's depression and everything associated with this, parents are more able to be in touch with their son's or daughter's distress and struggles, and better able to act effectively and in a considered way.

LOOKING TO THE FUTURE IN THE TREATMENT OF DEPRESSION IN ADOLESCENTS

Josie made good use of therapy, and by the end of the 28 sessions of therapy she no longer met diagnostic criteria for depression. Her scores on the Mood and Feelings Questionnaire[57] had changed from 41 (well above the clinical cutoff point) to 26 (just below it). She was more optimistic about life and had plans for the future.

Josie seemed relieved to find containment in her relationship with her therapist—someone who could reflect, make sense of nonverbal communication, and really hear and validate her emotional experiences. As her mood improved she found her own voice and became able to come to therapy alone. Toward the end of therapy Josie started to wear bright and then later feminine clothes, which suggested the beginning of adopting a more sexual feminine identity. She developed deeper same-sex friendships, although she still expressed fear about intimate relationships and a fear of abandonment. A similar fear was also expressed in her relationship with her therapist during the ending period of treatment. During the last phase of therapy, Josie was able to see the effect of her mother's past on her mother. As she did so she gained some emotional distance ("it's about her life, not about me") and individuation began. She also started to see school as a possible place for her development and future, although she needed a lot of support from the adults around her to return, and when treatment ended her school attendance was still erratic.

For Josie's parents, Michelle and David, the parent work enabled some emotional containment of their pain, and some differentiation of their own needs from those of Josie and her siblings. This process led to a lessening of their propensity to project unbearable anxieties, needs, and conflicts onto their children, and a greater capacity to support Josie with her own development.

Future Directions for Research on the Psychodynamic Treatment of Depression in Adolescence

As the authors have tried to illustrate in this article, psychodynamic psychotherapy can be a powerful intervention for depressed young people, especially those for whom depression is a marker of broader difficulties in negotiating the adolescent process. Although outcomes research in child and adolescent psychodynamic psychotherapy is still in its infancy, there is a growing body of empirical evidence to show the effectiveness of such an approach,[5] and there are several ongoing studies that also aim to throw more light on the elements of psychodynamic therapy with adolescents that may promote change (eg, Slonim and colleagues[58]).

The work by Blatt and colleagues[25,37] on adult depression is important because it not only begins to provide empirical support for certain subtypes of depression related to key psychodynamic features, it also relates these to therapeutic mechanisms that may help us as clinicians to know what kind of help is needed by different people with different kinds of psychological vulnerability to depression. Within the IMPACT study, psychodynamic patterns specific to adolescents suffering from depression will be systematically investigated to deepen our understanding of adolescent depression itself, and increase our understanding of how psychodynamic treatment can be most effective. The authors plan to use the Adolescent Psychotherapy Q-Set,[59] for example, to investigate the patterns of therapeutic interaction that emerge in different treatments, so that one can begin to relate certain psychodynamic patterns with therapeutic processes.

There is still a great deal to learn about adolescent depression, and much that can be learned about what are the most effective interventions to promote long-term recovery. We need to understand in more complex terms the multifaceted nature of adolescent depression, so as to unravel how those complex dynamics interact with particular therapeutic interactions and techniques. It is anticipated that the ongoing IMPACT study[4] will provide further opportunity to empirically investigate the mechanisms of change in psychodynamic psychotherapy with depressed adolescents, as well as an opportunity to investigate the experience of young people and their families receiving psychodynamic therapy (Midgley N, Target M. IMPACT: my experience—overcoming depression: Young peoples' experience of psychotherapy. 2011. Submitted for publication). Such studies will help us to develop a greater understanding of how psychodynamic therapy can help young people like Josie, and make a real contribution to the emotional well-being of depressed adolescents.

REFERENCES

1. World Health Organization. World health report. Geneva (Switzerland): World Health Organization; 2000.
2. Rudolph K, Klein D. Exploring depressive personality traits in youth: origins, correlates and developmental consequences. Dev Psychopathol 2009;21: 1155–80.
3. Jonsson U, Bohman H, von Knorring L, et al. Mental health outcome of long-term and episodic adolescent depression: 15-year follow-up of a community sample. J Affect Disord 2010;130(3):395–404.
4. Goodyer I, Tsancheva S, Byford S, et al. Improving mood with psychoanalytic and cognitive behavioural therapies (IMPACT): a pragmatic effectiveness superiority trial to investigate whether specialised psychological treatment reduces the risk for relapse in adolescents with moderate to severe unipolar depression: study protocol for a randomised controlled trial. Trials 2011;12(1):175.
5. Midgley N, Kennedy E. Psychodynamic psychotherapy for children and adolescents: a critical review of the evidence base. J Child Psychother 2011;37(3): 1–29.
6. Muratori F, Picchi L, Casella C, et al. Efficacy of brief dynamic psychotherapy for children with emotional disorders. Psychother Psychosom 2002;71(1): 28–38.
7. Muratori F, Picchi L, Bruni G, et al. A two-year follow-up of psychodynamic psychotherapy for internalizing disorders in children. J Am Acad Child Adolesc Psychiatry 2003;42(3):331–9.
8. Target M, Fonagy P. The efficacy of psycho-analysis for children with emotional disorders. J Am Acad Child Adolesc Psychiatry 1994;33(3):361–71.
9. Horn H, Geiser-Elze A, Reck C, et al. Efficacy of short term psychotherapy for children and adolescents with depression. Prax Kinderpsychol Kinderpsychiatr 2005;54(7):578–97.
10. Trowell J, Joffe I, Campbell J, et al. Childhood depression: a place for psychotherapy. An outcome study comparing individual psychodynamic psychotherapy and family therapy. Eur Child Adolesc Psychiatry 2007;16:157–67.
11. Trowell J, Miles G, editors. Childhood depression: a place for psychotherapy. London: Karnac; 2011.
12. Leichsenring F, Rabung S, Leibing E. The efficacy of short-term psychodynamic psychotherapy in specific psychiatric disorders: a meta-analysis. Arch Gen Psychiatry 2004;61:1208–16.
13. Leichsenring F, Rabung S. Effectiveness of long-term psychodynamic psychotherapy. JAMA 2008;300(13):1551–65.

14. de Maat S, de Jonghe F, Schoevers R, et al. The effectiveness of long-term psychoanalytic therapy: a systematic review of empirical studies. Harv Rev Psychiatry 2009;17(1):1–23.
15. Shedler J. The efficacy of psychodynamic psychotherapy. Am Psychol 2010; 65(2):98–109.
16. Malhi G, Adams D, Porter R, et al. Clinical practice recommendations for depression. Acta Psychiatr Scand 2009;119(Suppl 439):8–26.
17. de Maat S, Dekker J, Schoevers R, et al. Short term psychodynamic supportive psychotherapy, antidepressants, and their combination in the treatment of major depression: a mega-analysis based on three randomized clinical trials. Depress Anxiety 2008;25:565–74.
18. Abbass A, Town J, Driessen E. The efficacy of short-term psychodynamic psychotherapy for depressive disorders with comorbid personality disorders. Psychiatry 2011;74(1):61–74.
19. Freud S. Mourning and melancholia. In: Strachey J, editor. The standard edition of the complete psychological works of Sigmund Freud, vol. 14. London: Hogarth Press; 1917. p. 237–58.
20. Abraham K. A short study of the development of the libido, viewed in the light of the mental disorders. In: Abraham K, editor. Selected papers on psychoanalysis. London: Hogarth Press; 1927. p. 418–501.
21. Klein M. Mourning and its relation to manic-depressive states 1940. In: Klein M, editor. The writings of Melanie Klein, vol. 1. London: Hogarth; 1975. p. 344–69.
22. Bleichmar H. Some sub-types of depression and their implications for psychoanalytic treatment. Int J Psychoanal 1996;77:935–61.
23. Kernberg O. Borderline conditions and pathological narcissism. New York: Jason Aronson; 1975.
24. Kohut H. The restoration of the self. New York: Int Univ Press; 1977.
25. Blatt S. Contribution of psychoanalysis to the understanding and treatment of depression. J Am Psychoanal Assoc 1998;46:722–52.
26. Freud A. Normality and pathology in childhood: assessments of development. London: Karnac Books; 1996.
27. Erikson E. Childhood and Society. New York: W.W. Norton & Co; 1950.
28. Blos P. The second individuation process of adolescence. Psychoanal Study Child 1967;22:162–86.
29. Laufer M, Laufer E. Adolescent disturbance and breakdown. Harmondsworth (London): Penguin; 1975.
30. Rustin M. The psychology of depression in young adolescents: a psychoanalytic view of origins, inner workings and implications. Psychoanal Psychother 2009;23:3.
31. Bifulco A, Brown G, Harris T. Childhood loss of parent, lack of adequate parental care and adult depression: a replication. J Affect Disord 1987;12:115–28.
32. Gretton A. The wake-up call of adolescence: time-limited clinical work with three young people. In: Trowell J, Miles G, editors. Childhood depression: a place for psychotherapy. London: Karnac; 2011. p. 33–56.
33. Rhode M. Some reflections on the individual therapy: themes and interventions. In: Trowell J, Miles G, editors. Childhood depression: a place for psychotherapy. London: Karnac; 2011. p. 25–136.
34. Busch F, Rudden M, Shapiro T, editors. Psychodynamic treatment of depression. Washington, DC: American Psychiatric Publishing; 2004.
35. NICE. Depression in children and young people: identification and management in primary, community and secondary care. London: National Institute for Health and Clinical Excellence; 2005.

36. Ritvo RZ. Dynamic psychotherapy for the treatment of depression in youth. In: Rey JM, Birmaher B, editors. Treating child and adolescent depression. Philadelphia: Lippincott Williams & Wilkins; 2009. p. 140–50.
37. Luyten P, Blatt S. Psychodynamic treatment of depression. Psychiatr Clin North Am 2012;35(1):111–29.
38. Christogiorgos S, Stavrou E, Widdershoven-Zerkavi M, et al. Brief psychodynamic psychotherapy in adolescent depression: two case studies. In: Trowell J, Miles G, editors. Childhood depression: a place for psychotherapy. London: Karnac; 2011. p. 89–109.
39. Winnicott DW. Therapeutic consultations in child psychiatry. London: Hogarth and Institute of Psychoanalysis; 1972.
40. Lanyado M. Brief psychotherapy and therapeutic consultations: how much therapy is 'good enough'? In: Lanyado M, Horne A, editors. Handbook of child and adolescent psychotherapy. London: Routledge; 1999. p. 233–46.
41. Bion WR. A theory of thinking. Int J Psychoanal 1962;43:328–32.
42. Klein M. Notes on some schizoid mechanisms. Int J Psychoanal 1946;27:99–110.
43. Ogden T. Projective identification and psychotherapeutic technique. New York: Jason Aronson; 1982.
44. Pick IB. Working through in the countertransference. Int J Psychoanal 1985;66: 157–66.
45. Casement P. On learning from the patient. London: Routledge; 1985.
46. O'Shaughnessy E. What is a clinical fact? Int J Psychoanal 1994;75:939–47.
47. Heimann P. On countertransference. Int J Psychoanal 1950;31:81–4.
48. Bowlby J. The nature of the child's tie to his mother. Int J Psychoanal 1958;39:350.
49. Bowlby J. Attachment. In: Attachment and loss, vol. 1. New York: Basic Books; 1982 (Original work published 1969).
50. Bion WR. Elements of psychoanalysis. London: Heinemann; 1963.
51. Graham P, Hughes C. So young, so sad, so listen. London: Gaskell, Royal College of Psychiatrists; 2005.
52. Goodyer IM. The depressed child and adolescent. United Kingdom: Cambridge: Cambridge University Press; 2000.
53. Rustin M. Dialogues with parents. J Child Psychother 1998;24(2):233–52.
54. Tsintias J, Boethious S, Hallerfors B, et al, editors. Work with parents: psychoanalytic psychotherapy with children and adolescents. London: Karnac; 2000.
55. Miles G. The work with the parents alongside individual therapy with the children/young people: present and absent parents. In: Trowell J, Miles G, editors. Childhood depression: a place for psychotherapy. London: Karnac; 2011. p. 110–24.
56. Slade A. Parental reflective functioning: an introduction. Attach Hum Dev 2005; 7(3):269–81.
57. Daviss WB, Birmaher B, Melhem NA, et al. Criterion validity of the Mood and Feelings Questionnaire for depressive episodes in clinic and non-clinic subjects. J Child Psychol Psychiatry 2006;47(9):927–34.
58. Slonim DA, Shefler G, Gvirsman SD, et al. Changes in rigidity and symptoms among adolescents in psychodynamic psychotherapy. Psychother Res 2011; 21(6):685697.
59. Bychkova T, Hillman S, Midgley N, et al. The psychotherapy process with adolescents: preliminary comparisons between different therapeutic modalities using the Adolescent Psychotherapy Q-Set. J Child Psychother 2011;37(3):327–48.

Treatment of Anxiety in Children and Adolescents

Using Child and Adolescent Anxiety Psychodynamic Psychotherapy

Gabrielle Silver, MD*, Theodore Shapiro, MD, Barbara Milrod, MD

KEYWORDS

- Anxiety • Behavioral inhibition
- Child and adolescent psychodynamic psychotherapy • Phobia

KEY POINTS

- As new developmental tasks emerge in childhood, anxiety can miscarry and become anxiety disorders, severe and/or persistent, and can interfere with normal developmental tasks.
- In a psychoanalytic frame, anxiety can be understood in part as representing a "compromise formation." A compromise formation represents a psychological compromise between unacceptable or ambivalent wishes and defense mechanisms in response to those wishes.
- Child and adolescent psychodynamic psychotherapy is a manualized, time-limited psychodynamic psychotherapy with twice-weekly sessions, for children ages 8 to 16 years old with primary *Diagnostic and Statistical Manual of Mental Disorders* (fourth edition, text revision): generalized anxiety disorder, social phobia, or separation anxiety disorder. The therapeutic relationship is designed to help the child improve his or her capacity to reflect and better investigate and understand symptoms by beginning to articulate and explore underlying psychological meanings associated with them.

WHAT IS ANXIETY?

Anxiety is a universal human experience. Phenomenologically, it can comprise features of autonomic arousal, a subjective experience of tachycardia, increased respiration, and an acute sense of danger and dread. Human anxiety is closely related to mammalian fears and can be an inborn response to stimuli that the organism will actively attempt to avoid via flight or freezing.[1] Developmentally anxiety is adaptive and useful, alerting the child to the perceived threat of danger. Anxiety is also elicited

Department of Child and Adolescent Psychiatry, NYP Weill Cornell Medical College, 525 East 68th Street, Box 140, New York, NY 10065, USA
* Corresponding author.
E-mail address: ghs2001@med.cornell.edu

Child Adolesc Psychiatric Clin N Am 22 (2013) 83–96
http://dx.doi.org/10.1016/j.chc.2012.08.005 **childpsych.theclinics.com**
1056-4993/13/$ – see front matter

Key Abbreviations: Anxiety	
CAMS	Child-Adolescent Anxiety Multimodal Study
CAPP	Child and adolescent psychodynamic psychotherapy
CBT	Cognitive-behavioral therapy
GAD	Generalized anxiety disorder
OCD	Obsessive-compulsive disorder
PD	Panic disorder
PFPP	Panic focused psychodynamic psychotherapy
PTSD	Posttraumatic stress disorder
RF	Reflective functioning

as a response to ruptured attachments. Separation anxiety is but the first of a sequence of danger signals during development. However, as new developmental tasks emerge in childhood, anxiety can miscarry and become anxiety disorders, severe and/or persistent, and can interfere with normal developmental tasks.

Anxiety disorders are the most frequent mental disorders among children and can cause substantial impairment in school, family relationships, and social functioning.[2–4] Childhood anxiety disorders most commonly present first as separation anxiety and specific phobias, followed by the onset of social phobia.[5,6] There is evidence that inhibited temperament is related to the development of anxiety disorders.[5,6] The slow-to-warm-up, cautious, and hyperalert stance of children with anxious temperaments, in its most extreme form, with behavioral inhibition, suggests a lower threshold for anxiety in response to environmental stressors.[7,8] Behavioral inhibition is operationally measured by cautious exploration of novel environments and even an aversion to novelty. Anxiety in adulthood is commonly preceded by anxiety in childhood.[4,9,10] One goal of early ascertainment and treatment of anxiety in childhood and adolescence is to try to limit the development of mood and anxiety disorders later in life.

Diagnoses classified as Anxiety Disorders in the *Diagnostic and Statistical Manual of Mental Disorders*, fourth edition, text revision (DSM-IV-TR)[11] include: generalized anxiety disorder (GAD), specific phobia, agoraphobia, panic disorder (PD), social phobia, posttraumatic stress disorder (PTSD), and obsessive-compulsive disorder (OCD). Evolving neurobiological understanding, coupled with overlapping characteristics of the current diagnoses and the heterogeneity of signs and symptoms among anxiety disorders, has provided a rationale to realign these categories in DSM-V such that PTSD and OCD will be presented as distinct categories from the other anxiety disorders.[12,13]

Nonpsychodynamic Treatment Approaches to the Treatment of Anxiety

Nonpharmacologic treatments for childhood anxiety are frequently preferred by children and their parents, and are recommended for the many youth with anxiety disorders who either do not respond well to medications or develop adverse events from antianxiety medication.[14–16] The largest study of note in childhood anxiety disorders, the Child-Adolescent Anxiety Multimodal Study (CAMS), demonstrated that children with anxiety disorders respond to cognitive-behavioral therapy (CBT) and pharmacologic interventions, and that CBT and their combination were superior to placebo.[17] In this randomized controlled trial conducted across 6 sites, 488 children aged 7 to 17 with primary DSM-IV diagnoses of social anxiety disorder (SAD), GAD, or social phobia were assigned to receive 14 sessions of CBT (based on the Coping CAT Program[18] adapted for the subjects' age and duration of the study),[18,19] sertraline or a combination of sertraline and CBT, or a placebo for 12 weeks. Roughly 50% of both sertraline and CBT-alone treated groups were found to be much improved or very much improved on the Clinical Global Impression of Improvement ($P<.001$), in contrast to 80% of those treated with the combination ($P<.001$) and 23.7% treated with placebo.

Psychodynamic Approaches to the Treatment of Anxiety

Psychodynamic psychotherapy has been used to treat anxious children since the 1940s but has yet to be systematically tested in children. In a psychoanalytic frame, anxiety can be understood in part as representing a "compromise formation." A compromise formation represents a psychological compromise between unacceptable or ambivalent wishes and defense mechanisms in response to those wishes. The emotional pressure of both the unacceptable wishes and their defense leads to symptoms. Defense mechanisms, which are themselves unconscious psychological processes, protect the individual from the psychological danger arising from unacceptable wishes and fantasies. If the defenses fail (ie, the child becomes aware of the depth of his rage at his mother, for example), the child experiences overwhelming anxiety. **Box 1** outlines a developmental progression of anxiety-provoking psychological situations that can engender these psychological processes that trigger symptoms of anxiety.

A symptom-focused manualized psychoanalytic psychotherapy, panic-focused psychodynamic psychotherapy (PFPP), was found to have efficacy for adults with primary PD with or without agoraphobia.[20] Child and adolescent anxiety psychodynamic psychotherapy (CAPP), the symptom-focused manualized form of psychodynamic therapy the authors have been testing in a small open clinical trial, has been adapted to younger developmental age groups from PFPP.[21]

CHILD AND ADOLESCENT ANXIETY PSYCHODYNAMIC PSYCHOTHERAPY MANUAL

CAPP is a manualized, time-limited psychodynamic psychotherapy with twice-weekly sessions, for children ages 8 to 16 years old with primary DSM-IV-TR: GAD, social

Box 1
Anxiety provoked by unconscious and ambivalent aspects of common childhood dilemmas

Unacceptable Ideas/Wishes Evoked By:

- Life events such as birth of sibling or loss of exclusive hold on parent
- Family relationships, such as parental discord, abuse
- Triangular allegiances and conflicts in family
- Meanings of events based on perceptual distortion and immature interpretation (eg, being trapped in an elevator and fearing never to see mother again)

Common Dynamisms Underlying Youth Anxiety:

- Fear of separation from attachment figures, ambivalence about autonomy, conflated with fears of loss
- Difficulty experiencing/acknowledging anger and/or ambivalence toward attachment figures
- Sexual conflicts as sexual identity emerges (eg, unacceptable masturbation fantasies)
- Guilty self punishment through the experience of anxiety symptoms per se

Normative Developmental Pressures—Stage-Related Equilibria, Transitioning from Home to Community, Cognitive Maturity

- 8 to 11 years old: latency search for mastery over intellectual and physical skills; phase-related righteousness (harsh superego)
- 12 to 16 years old: early adolescent search for independent identity and further mastery over preferred endeavors. New integration of bodily sensations, anatomy, sexuality

phobia, or separation anxiety disorder. CAPP is made up of 20 to 24 sessions divided into 3 phases (**Box 2**). The therapeutic relationship is designed to help the child improve his or her capacity to reflect, and better investigate and understand symptoms by beginning to articulate and explore underlying psychological meanings associated with them. Symptoms include the physiologic (autonomic) signs of anxiety such as shortness of breath, sweating, and shaking, as well as the associated cognitive accompaniments such as overwhelming fear and paralysis. Throughout the therapy, the therapist and patient work to better understand and articulate the underlying psychological conflicts that engender the anxiety (**Box 3**).

This approach makes the basic assumption that symptoms carry specific psychological meaning, and that this can be ascertained through the exploration of personal fantasies and meanings connected with the anxiety. In the early phase of CAPP, the therapist develops a working psychodynamic formulation that itself is psychodynamic (ie, subject to change as more information is gathered) about the psychological

Box 2
Therapeutic process and strategies

Phase 1

- History from family (context)
- Developing alliance as narrative of symptoms unfolds in context of life events
- Therapist listening: tentative psychodynamic formulations
- Primary dynamisms identified
- Present dynamism to patient, focusing on meaning of continuing dialogue where it fits
- There is a continuous focus on anxiety symptoms by the therapist whether the patient brings it up or not

Phase 2

- Continue dialogue: patient sets focus/topics
- Anxiety focus
- Therapist finds redundant expositions, questions and clarifies/applies psychodynamic focus, repeatedly interpreting
- Patient begins to be reflective and self-observing about anxiety
- Loosening the fixity of reaction patterns: opens inquiry for new responses
- Patient considers other examples of how dynamisms effect anxiety/behavior
- Therapist reinforces reflective function, accenting tendency to repeat

Phase 3

- Commonly punctuated by anxiety symptom rearousal
- Demonstration of transference as recurrence of separation anxiety and difficulty with ambivalence and rage
- Revisit with family of younger patients/crises
- Repetition and working through dynamism discovered
- Reinforce reflection and newly established flexibility of response
- Advocate for new open behavior, diminishing tendency to withdraw/fall into repetitive patterns

Box 3
CAPP treatment overview

A. History from family and child
   a. 12 to 16 years old: at least one meeting with parents and adolescent. Delineate the role of anxiety in the family and the place of the adolescent's symptoms in the family
   b. 8 to 11 years old: 1 to 2 meetings with parents held without the child before treatment, then again throughout the course of the therapy as needed
B. Develop a specific psychodynamic formulation of meaning of anxiety symptoms
   a. Reflective functioning: awaken psychological curiosity
   b. Alternative meanings offered through interpretation of fantasies
   c. Developmental orientation
C. Talk/play (depending on age of patient): learn from the child what his/her point of view is, help the child conceptualize that he/she can understand what might be going on in the mind of another through imagining how he/she might feel in a given situation
   a. 8 to 10 years old: more activity driven (play and drawing)
   b. 11 to 16 years old: more verbal dialogue (play or drawing if necessary)
D. Interpret commonly appearing defenses
   a. Denial, turning passive into active, projection, regression, and isolation of affect
E. Rapid communication of patient's conflicts, verbally and respectfully: connecting anxiety symptoms, fantasies, affects, and interactions within the context of therapeutic relationship
F. Careful listening to patient reactions (modification of formulation) (feeling understood)
G. Discovery of unconscious fantasies through daydreams, dream, play, which can be expressed, tolerated, and treated as openings for inquiry
H. Connecting fantasies directly to the anxiety symptoms (loosening the entrenched constellations leading to maladaptations)
I. Fantasies and defenses reconsidered in light of present needs and coping abilities, with the new realization that they are anachronisms from earlier phases of life and can be dispensed with or altered so that the patient can move to the appropriate developmental stage

meaning of the anxiety symptoms. Later in the therapy, the therapist progressively returns to repetitive examples of dynamisms in the child's life and to the transference to reveal and further develop this evolving formulation and permit the child to witness the repetitive occurrence of the same psychological constellation. This process leads to symptom relief through various mechanisms (**Table 1**).

Reflective functioning (RF) is a proposed mechanism through which psychodynamic therapy works. RF is a way of codifying the ability to understand one's own mind and other people's minds. This "reflectiveness" develops when the caregiver's mindfulness about a child's mental state allows the child to develop capacities of self regulation, and the ability to envision and think about mental states in oneself and, therefore, the capacity for empathy and intimacy. When RF improves the patient's insight improves.[22]

Treatment begins with history gathering. With younger children, meetings take place with parents separately; developing and maintaining an alliance with parents is important. Individual therapy with the child includes a safe and cooperative environment where the focus is on the child's current experience and anxiety.

Table 1
Relationship between psychodynamic theory and interventions for anxiety in CAPP

Anxiety Disorder Features	Psychodynamic Theory in CAPP	Target Symptoms and CAPP Strategies
Social phobia	Extreme self consciousness and fears of embarrassing oneself are linked to conflicted wishes to be the center of attention and laced with guilt and self punishment; normal desire for attention feels unacceptably aggressive	Explore defenses against wishes to stand out, conflicted patients' overly critical evaluation of others as entrée to connections with uncomfortable competitive wishes and conflicted, unacceptable aggression. This raises SSRF
GAD	Extreme inability to relax, hypervigilance, and dread of many life situations arises from conflicts related to personal meanings of curiosity and exploration of new and novel situations; normal curiosity and desire for exploration is associated with feeling dangerously out of control and overwhelmed	Focus on terror of internal urges, including aggression and desire for autonomy. Emerging fantasies actively connected with symptoms and persistence of anxiety. This raises SSRF
Separation anxiety	Severe, developmentally inappropriate separation distress arises from conflicts between normal strivings for autonomy and concerns about hurting or infuriating the emotionally needed parent. Clinging to parent leads to anger at parent and self; normal strivings for autonomy are associated with feeling unacceptably lonely and frighteningly rejecting of the parent	Explore transference, an emotionally vibrant paradigm for understanding and altering separation fears. Intensity (twice a week) and brevity (for 12 weeks) are key CAPP aspects making emotional significance of termination central to the final third of treatment. This raises SSRF
Anxiety reestablishing age-appropriate autonomy, common to these disorders	Conflicts and fears about normal autonomy (ie, growing wish to manage by oneself, curiosity and independence) common in SP, GAD, and SAD patients emerge in transference. Assertiveness (seeking attention, exploring and attempts at independence), perceived as destructive anger, creating conflict	CAPP focus on transference highlights conflicts about autonomy, especially as incorporated into fantasies of bodily harm; sense of inadequacy is experienced as physical anxiety and symptoms

(*continued on next page*)

Table 1
(continued)

Anxiety Disorder Features	Psychodynamic Theory in CAPP	Target Symptoms and CAPP Strategies
Comorbid major depression-when present	Conflicted aggression leads to guilt and negative self evaluation, depressive symptoms, and somatic anxiety	CAPP focus on conflicted aggression detoxifies and helps patient redirect it, improving autonomous function and assertion. Mitigates guilt, with improvement in autonomy, negative views of self improvement

Abbreviations: CAPP, child and adolescent psychodynamic psychotherapy; GAD, generalized anxiety disorder; SAD, social anxiety disorder; SP, social phobia; SSRF, symptom specific reflective functioning.

For older children and adolescents, encouraging parental support while fostering developmentally appropriate autonomy is central to the success of therapy. Maintaining an alliance with the family can be essential to engaging the child, particularly at moments of emotional turmoil. Throughout the course of treatment, the therapist first develops a working formulation about underlying meanings of the patient's anxiety, then refines it, to connect current crises that emerge (eg, child stops going to school, has panic attack on bus, and so forth) with underlying anxiety psychodynamics. Transference is explored to the extent that it is possible in the context of a time-limited psychotherapy. Core anxiety psychodynamics (wishes, adaptation to reality, atoning for guilty transgressions) are identified across various areas of the patient's life. Emphasis is placed on ways in which the child's coping style may have been adaptive for the child earlier, and yet is not serving him or her in current circumstances. This approach helps the child develop more appropriate, less dysfunctional mechanisms for handling emotional conflicts.

In the latter part of therapy, termination must be discussed actively by the therapist. This period is often a symptomatic time, during which primary conflicts about being able to act autonomously, accelerated by the experience of ambivalent anger about separation from the therapist as termination is approached, necessarily emerge in the therapeutic relationship. This situation can provide the opportunity for the child to experience these conflicts directly in the room with the therapist.

THE CASE OF MAX

Max was a 16-year-old boy of high academic achievement, from a professional family, who presented with symptoms of GAD (6/8), social phobia (5/8), and dysthymia (4/8) on the Anxiety Disorders Interview Scale (ADIS) for Child and Parent, with a score of 22 on the Pediatric Anxiety Rating Scale—Revised (PARS-R). Max's presenting symptoms included generalized anxiety and worry about academic performance, social acceptance, and heightened conflict with his mother. He was very anxious with peers, socially inhibited in the classroom, and had difficulty sleeping and fatigue. His mother was concerned about his waning school performance, lack of initiative, and poor response to limit setting. Max felt he was doing "OK" in school, and wished his parents would "leave him alone."

Max's family was beset by the economic downturn and a recent apartment move. Max had suffered injuries preventing him from playing sports, involvement with which was central to his identity. In addition, his parents did not approve of his new girlfriend.

During the first phase of treatment, rapport was easily established. Although he was "not used to this," the therapist helped him express feelings and experiences. Max explained, in his quiet manner, that being quiet helped him manage at home where he perceived his mother to be "the dictator." The therapist noted that it appeared that he and his "father both seemed to have similar responses" to his mother. The patient acknowledged, "I kind of copied him..." By the next session the patient's silence provided an opportunity for the therapist to interpret Max's routine manner of handling social interactions, repeated with him, in the transference. The initial dynamism explored was suppression of both anger and expression of age-related assertiveness.

During the second phase of treatment Max's conflict avoidance emerged during intercurrent crises: escalating active conflict with his parents around weekend activities. The now more expressive and angry Max heightened parental concern that "things are exploding." In session Max reported that his "parents are the source of my anxiety." The therapist pointed out that Max needed to find the source of his feelings and behaviors outside himself rather than within as conflicted wishes. His worried parents called to see if medication was not called for. At the same time as increasing "storms" were reported by Max's parents there was "calm" during sessions, combined with Max missing/forgetting sessions and long silences in the room. As the crisis with his parents resolved, Max began to emphasize his improved school performance and a return to sports. The brevity of treatment can lead to an acting out of therapeutic health that needs to be interpreted.

The treatment entered the termination phase, and Max reported feeling "a lot better." There was a mild reemergence of original symptoms of fatigue, insomnia, conflicts at home, and avoidance of social interactions. During this phase the subject of the loss of his therapist was highlighted and discussed. Max's anxiety remitted with therapy. On termination his PARS-R score was 12; on the ADIS he had lost his diagnoses for GAD and social phobia, and dysthymia was 4/8.

Discussion

This case represents an example of a teen living in a relatively supportive environment where the developmentally appropriate conflict between his desire for greater autonomy and the acceptance of developmentally necessary levels of dependence on parents (financial, educational, and so forth) was expressed in anxiety symptoms. Max did several things that augmented his dependence (ie, his passivity, encouraging his mother to step in) and obscured awareness of feelings by "checking out" regarding his mother. His unrealistic expectations and attitudes toward his current developmental situation and the emergent anger and resentment frightened him, but he quickly bypassed evidence of this suppressed rage with anxiety.

He was enraged and guilty toward his father too for being so passive in dealing with his demanding, intrusive mother, yet identified most with him in his passive role in the family. He unconsciously punished himself and his family for gratification of his unconscious passive wishes. Max's maladaptive use of passivity as solution to conflict with his mother and sister contrasted with his unconscious wishes for success and triumph over his parents. During treatment and based on a new relationship that permitted expression of emergent feelings, he was able to articulate and tolerate some of these age-appropriate wishes and also explore his feelings in the transference. He increasingly engaged with family, and sought greater developmentally congruent independence and success in his endeavors. The new consideration of feelings from within rather than reaction to external behavior of others is a hallmark of a psychodynamic approach. CBT or other approaches that are based on response prevention or fear appraisal would not engender the reflection necessary to reappraise the sources of anxiety and the defenses against inner drives and affects. The experience of affects previously suppressed permitted age-appropriate developmental advances as well.

MARC: CAPP FOR A COMPLEX CASE

Marc was a 12-year-old seventh grader at a parochial day school who lived with his mother and stepfather. He presented with escalating anxiety in school and in other public arenas. He was encouraged by his school counselor to enter the CAPP study. Mother was concerned that he did not want to invite friends home, staying both physically and emotionally on "the fringe of things." During wrestling practice he stayed in an adjoining gym with her until practice started, and he sat away from other teammates when not wrestling. Marc never raised his hand in class, and he became extremely anxious when tested or when there was a change in routine. Mother informed the therapist that as a small child Marc had had a little stuffed animal that he would suck on in times of stress, which his parents took away from him when he was age 8 or 9, at which point he developed a tic that looked like a sucking motion.

On presentation, mother described Marc as having tics at times of increased stress. He was so soft spoken that people would often ask him to speak up, and at other times because of his extreme reserve, cousins asked his mother if he was angry about something, which he always denied. Marc had been overweight, and lost 30 lb before presenting in an effort to meet athletic standards. He was uncomfortable eating in public, and worried that people were thinking "look at that fat pig eating that food."

At age 9 Marc had a grand mal seizure, but evaluation including electroencephalography was normal. For a short time after this he asked his mother to sleep with him, which she did for a month. Mother indicated that he sought proximity in whichever room she or his step-dad chose. Mother described him as overly sensitive with others, worrying that he was not liked or loved, and easily felt criticized or embarrassed. When he felt he was on display, such as the wrestling award ceremony, he became distraught and threw up. He refused to have a birthday party, and only enjoyed social events with his cousins. However, he was comfortable performing when he played the saxophone.

Mother and father separated when Marc was 4 years old, when they moved from the West Coast to New York City. Marc's biological father, a fireman, suffered from bipolar disorder and was abusive, "just not a good person." Mother is in the Navy and often on duty. Marc was intermittently raised by his maternal grandparents when his mother was deployed to distant war zones every 2 to 3 years. (She had been deployed for 4 months on when he was 2 and 4, and when he was 10 she was overseas for a year.)

When Marc began CAPP he scored 26 on the PARS-R,[23] and on the ADIS[24] he was diagnosed with social phobia (6/8), SAD (4/8), and GAD (5/8). His mother was scheduled to leave for duty in a war zone toward the end of the scheduled 24 sessions. Marc had seen his father during the summers until 4 years before the start of treatment, when his father fell out of touch. The Christmas before treatment started, mother contacted father to tell him to call his son and he told her, "just tell him I called and sent my love." Father was in another relationship after the divorce from Marc's mother, and had a daughter with whom Marc has had some contact and whom he called his sister. Father currently sees neither child.

In New York City, Marc is the eldest of 9 cousins and spends much of his free time with them and his 5 maternal aunts and their husbands. In addition, he has a relationship with his paternal grandparents, and with his stepfather's family.

In the first phase of treatment, Marc was very quiet. He initially told the therapist much of the same information that he and his mother reported to the diagnostician, but soon after that he became nearly silent. The therapist's initial formulation included the impression that Marc was stalled developmentally, and acted as if he were around 4 or 5 years old. At that age he had been separated from his father, and had witnessed his father physically and emotionally abuse his mother. Marc was thought to have unresolved conflicts about what it might mean to be a man, as well as a great deal of fear about losing his mother, who frequently disappeared to her naval duties and who was at realistic risk of death. The therapist interpreted Marc's silence as a way to avoid painful and unacceptable feelings of anger that he felt toward his mother and biological father for leaving him. Because he could not tolerate the rage he felt for his mother, the woman he most loved and on whom he was dependent, or the rage at the father who could abandon him, he resorted to silence as a defense against what he felt would be a dangerous rage, and overwhelming sadness. This constellation was addressed as the first central dynamism; the therapist told Marc that a secondary gain of silence was the possibility of denying the existence of such feelings altogether. He tried to protect himself from these feelings by literally not giving them a voice. During an early session he talked about not wanting to go to the camp his mother had planned for him because he wanted to go to wrestling camp, but he literally could not tell her. First, the therapist interpreted his anger about his mother making decisions for him without consulting him, and then highlighted his contribution to this situation by not speaking up for fear of making her angry and the perceived threat of abandonment.

After this interpretation he uncharacteristically approached his mother about camp. He also began telling the therapist about how his mother made him feel like a Mama's boy because "she treats me like a 6-year-old." He described mother's demanding too loudly that he put on his socks or drink his Gatorade in practice. The therapist then interpreted how he might have conflicting feelings, wanting to be a Mama's boy, and wanting to be more independent, but how very unfair it was that he has had less control because his mother has had to leave so many times and for such long periods of time, and that once again separation was looming ahead. Marc verbally rejected this interpretation, but for the next weeks he was much more talkative than he was during the first phase of treatment. He began discussing some of his frustrations and experiences in school and at home. He began to seem less anxious and more irritable.

In the middle phase of treatment Marc spoke more spontaneously, and readily described interactions with friends and family. Mother prepared to leave and met with the therapist and Marc during one session. In that session she became tearful. In the following session, Marc and the therapist discussed how difficult it might be to express his anger with mother if he feared she might get weepy in response. During the sixth week of therapy, after a session in which he told the therapist that he hadn't wanted to come, he'd have "preferred to stay home and prepare for practice," he was able to describe how anxious he became about the matches, how unsure he was that he "will do the right thing." He described feeling strongly that he should be able to know all the moves expected and yet he found it "difficult to remember."

The therapist pointed out how hard he was on himself, how infrequently he allowed himself to be proud of himself, and how quick he was to experience himself as inadequate even when his shortcomings were shared by many of his peers; this led to a discussion of how fearful he was that strangers would think he was weird if he was reading a book about wrestling on the subway. The therapist highlighted Marc's sense that he had something very shameful about himself hidden, but dangerously ready to be discovered.

At the next session Marc disclosed what felt to him like a very big, bad secret, that his father was Moroccan (the therapist had not known this), and the therapist pointed out the possibility of whether he might be even more afraid of people knowing that his father was mentally ill and behaved so erratically. This notion was explored, and he admitted how afraid he was that people would know about his father. He secretly worried that this reflected on his having some hidden flaw or inadequacy. After this set of discussions, Marc engaged with friends with greater frequency and more openly. He began to wrestle more seriously, and experienced himself as a valued member of his team.

Early in the third phase of therapy, Marc talked a good deal about a plan he had to visit his biological father during the summer. He talked about his paternal family and their country life. In talking about them sometimes his voice broke from its usual monotone into a more expressive and brighter rhythm, but he would quickly catch himself. If the therapist brought his attention to this liveliness he denied it, and conversation would stall.

As per CAPP protocol, the therapist began talking with Marc about the treatment ending at the beginning of the third month. Soon after she did this, he fell silent again. This time, he did not hide his reluctance to come but told his grandparents that he didn't want to come. He also missed a few wrestling practices, and was sick and stayed home from school. Marc and the therapist discussed this reluctance to attend sessions in the context of how frequently he could not control the comings and goings of people dear to him, like his mother and father, and how terrible it must feel because he had had so many losses and separations in his life. More importantly, he was being separated from his mother again for 3 to 4 months, and now the therapist too was going to leave him. He responded to these interpretations with relief.

As treatment ended, Marc increased his engagement with friends, even doing things he was not supposed to do in school and at home, testing limits for the first time. He began speaking up for himself, much to the relief and frustration of his parents and grandparents. One day he told the therapist that he had been running around with some of his friends in the staircase at school, and a few of them had waited for another friend and tripped him at the bottom of the stairs. This prank was one of a few he ever engaged in and had gotten into trouble for at school. The therapist said she wondered if he hadn't begun to more ably express aggression, but maybe it wasn't actually that boy he was angry at. He agreed but seemed pleased with himself that he had been part of the trouble instead of looking in from the outside and feeling like an outsider. At the time of termination his mother was deployed, and Marc was doing better in school and at home. His termination PARS-R was 13, and ADIS was GAD 4/8. He had lost his diagnoses of SAD and separation anxiety disorder on the ADIS.

Discussion

This study is a fairly representative case of a youth with anxiety presenting for treatment with evidence of severe, limiting anxiety, withdrawal, and a developmental derailment. This 12-year-old boy had experienced a severe trauma (abuse of his mother by his father, separation from both parents, divorce) at 4 years old, and presented with the defensive style and coping skills of a 4- to 5-year-old. The familial style of this military family was quite reserved, and Marc's preference to contain his feelings about his repeated losses interfered with his ability to develop a sense of safety and of an autonomous self. His conflicts about his own aggression toward and fear of his father left him unable to explore his own fantasies, feelings, or preferences, much less to be assertive about realizing them.

Because his conflicted need to be the center of his mother's attention was so frequently impossible to realize, he was not able to develop healthy self refection and a compassionate conscience. Through this brief anxiety-focused psychodynamic intervention his symptoms remitted, his reflective functioning improved, he developed the capacity to be increasingly and more age-appropriately assertive, and he overcame his sense of danger and inner prohibitions without threat of abandonment. His final evaluation revealed remission of his symptoms, as can be seen by his posttreatment scores.

The use of a psychodynamic approach in this treatment seemed apt given the complexity of his environment. He could not easily see that some of what he experienced derived from inner conflict. He was not accustomed to reflection and metacognitive exploration. The opening phases of a new relationship that encouraged exploration and expression permitted the elaboration of a primary dynamism to be confronted repeatedly. This sort of intervention was again apt because at each encounter new events could be absorbed into the ongoing exploration, and the boy felt he was understood and could consider his transference wishes.

Given his father's chronic and severe symptomatology and diagnosis of bipolar disorder, it is quite likely that this patient is biologically vulnerable to anxiety and mood dysregulation. Nonetheless, Marc demonstrably benefited from a time-limited, symptom-focused psychodynamic treatment. By treatment termination he began to behave and conceptualize himself in a more developmentally appropriate fashion, revealing that treatment is more than a reduction of symptoms.

SUMMARY: LOOKING TO THE FUTURE OF CAPP

Anxiety disorders are common among children, causing substantial impairment in school, family relationships, and social functioning. Given the evolving understanding that mood and anxiety disorders likely share neurobiological genetic vulnerability, and that childhood anxiety, temperamental disposition, and separation anxiety frequently precede adult anxiety and mood disorders, it behooves us to identify and offer a range of treatments for children who are suffering from these disorders. Pharmacotherapy is frequently not the treatment of choice. CBT is efficacious for youth anxiety, although excellent response rates attenuate over time.[16] Preliminary results of the CAPP protocol have been promising, with subjects experiencing significant, clinically meaningful improvements across all measured areas. As with the case examples, most subjects not only had symptom relief but also were able to advance in developmental experience and use their therapeutic experience reflectively. In conclusion, it may be beneficial to treat children and adolescents with anxiety disorders with symptom-focused, manualized psychodynamic psychotherapy, and once a sufficient pilot sample can be reported it should be replicated in a randomized controlled trial.

REFERENCES

1. Neuman ID, Wigger A, Kromer S, et al. Differential effects of periodic maternal separation on adult stress coping in a rat model of extremes in trait anxiety. Neuroscience 2005;132:867–77.
2. Anderson JC, Williams S. DSM-III disorders in preadolescent children. Arch Gen Psychiatry 1987;(44):69–76.

3. Rutter M. Isle of Wight revisited: twenty five years of child psychiatric epidemiology [special article]. J Am Acad Child Adolesc Psychiatry 1989;28: 633–53.
4. Beesdo K, Knappe S, Pine D. Anxiety and anxiety disorders in children and adolescents: Developmental issues and Implications for DSM-V. Psych Clin North Am 2009;32(3):483–524.
5. Kagan J, Reznick JS, Snidman N. Biological bases of childhood shyness. Science 1988;240:167–71.
6. Menin DS, Fresco DM, Heimberg RG, et al. Screening for social anxiety disorder in the clinical setting: using the Liebowitz Social Anxiety Scale. J Anxiety Disord 2002;16(6):661–73.
7. Biederman J, Rosenbaum JF, Bolduc-Murphy EA, et al. 3-year follow-up of children with and without behavioral inhibition. J Am Acad Child Adolesc Psychiatry 1993;32(4):814–21.
8. Rosenbaum JF, Biederman J, Gersten M, et al. Behavioral inhibition in children of parents with panic disorder and agoraphobia. A controlled study. Arch Gen Psychiatry 1988;45:463–70.
9. Ferdinand RF, Verhulst FC. Psychopathology from adolescence into young adulthood: an 8 year follow-up study. Am J Psychiatry 1995;152:1586–94.
10. Pine DS, Cohen P, Gurley D, et al. The risk for early adulthood anxiety and depressive disorders in adolescents with anxiety and depressive disorders. Arch Gen Psychiatry 1998;55:56–64.
11. Diagnostic and statistical manual of mental disorders. 4th edition, text revision: DSM-IV-TR. Washington, DC: American Psychiatric Association; 2000.
12. Rosen GM, Lilienfeld SO, Frueh C, et al. Reflections of PTSD's future in DSM-V. Br J Psychol 2010;197:343–4.
13. Beesdo K, Knappe S, Pine D. Anxiety and anxiety disorders in children and adolescents: developmental issues and implications for DSM V. Psychiatr Clin North Am 2009;32(3):483–524.
14. Warden D, Trivedi MH, Wisniewski SR, et al. Early adverse events and attrition in SSRI Treatment: a suicide assessment methodology study (SAMS) report. J Clin Psychopharmacol 2010;30(3):259–66.
15. Kisicki HA, Varley C. Efficacy and safety of antidepressant drug treatment in children and adolescents. Mol Psychiatry 2011. http://dx.doi.org/10.1038/mp.2011.150.
16. Ginsburg GS, Kendall PC, Sakolsky D, et al. Remission after acute treatment in children and adolescents with anxiety disorders: findings from the CAMS. J Consult Clin Psychol 2011;79(6):806–13.
17. Walkup JT, Albano AM, Piacentini J, et al. Cognitive behavior therapy, sertraline, or a combination in childhood anxiety. N Engl J Med 2008;359(26):2753–66.
18. Kendall PC, Hedtke KA. Coping CAT workbook. 2nd edition. Ardmore (PA): Workbook Publishing; 2006.
19. Kendall PC, Hedtke KA. Cognitive-behavior therapy for anxious children: therapist manual. 3rd edition. Ardmore (PA): Workbook Publishing; 2006.
20. Milrod B, Busch F, Cooper A, et al. Manual of panic—focused psychodynamic psychotherapy. Washington, DC: APA Press; 1997.
21. Milrod B, Leon AC, Busch FN, et al. A randomized controlled clinical trial of psychoanalytic psychotherapy for panic disorder. Am J Psychiatry 2007;164:265–72.
22. Bouchard MA, Target M, Lecours S, et al. Mentalization in adult attachment narratives; reflective functioning, mental states, and affect elaboration compared. Psychoanal Psychol 2008;25(1):47–66.

23. The Pediatric anxiety rating scale (PARS) development and psychometric properties. J Am Acad Child Adolesc Psychiatry 2002;41(9):1061–9.
24. Grills A, Ollendick T. Multiple informant agreement and the anxiety disorders interview schedule for parents and children. J Am Acad Child Adolesc Psychiatry 2003;42(1):30–40.

Eating Disorders in Adolescents

Review of Treatment Studies that Include Psychodynamically Informed Therapy

Ida Dancyger, PhD[a,b,*], Scott Krakower, DO[b,c],
Victor Fornari, MD[a,b]

KEYWORDS

- Eating disorder(s) • Psychodynamic • Anorexia nervosa • Bulimia nervosa
- Adolescents • Psychotherapy

KEY POINTS

- Eating disorders (EDs) in children and adolescents are serious psychiatric conditions often requiring a team approach, including medical monitoring, nutritional rehabilitation, family therapy, and individual psychotherapy.
- The psychotherapy evidence base is strongest for the Maudsley model of family therapy for youth with anorexia nervosa (AN) living at home and for cognitive behavioral therapy for adults and adolescents with bulimia nervosa (BN).
- In clinical practice, psychodynamic approaches represent an important component of the treatment for young people with EDs.
- Review of research studies of psychodynamically informed therapies for EDs suggests that further research into these treatments is warranted.

INTRODUCTION

Anorexia nervosa (AN) and bulimia nervosa (BN) in children and adolescents present as serious, complex medical-psychiatric problems that require a multimodal team approach. The research literature remains modest regarding the most effective treatment for children, adolescents, or adults with an eating disorder (ED). Cognitive-behavioral treatment (CBT) has the best evidence base as an intervention for BN.

The authors have nothing to disclose.
[a] Zucker Hillside Hospital, 75-59 263rd Street, Glen Oaks, NY 11004, USA; [b] Division of Child and Adolescent Psychiatry, Department of Psychiatry, Zucker Hillside Hospital, 75-59 263rd Street, Glen Oaks, NY 11004, USA; [c] Child and Adolescent Psychiatry, Hofstra North-Shore-LIJ School of Medicine, Hempstead, NY 11549-1000, USA
* Corresponding author. Division of Child and Adolescent Psychiatry, Department of Psychiatry, Zucker Hillside Hospital, 75-59 263rd Street, Glen Oaks, New York 11004.
E-mail address: ida.dancyger@gmail.com

Child Adolesc Psychiatric Clin N Am 22 (2013) 97–117
http://dx.doi.org/10.1016/j.chc.2012.08.006 **childpsych.theclinics.com**

Abbreviations: Eating Disorders	
AFT	Adolescent focused individual therapy
AN	Anorexia nervosa
BFST	Behavioral family systems therapy
BN	Bulimia nervosa
CAT	Cognitive analytic therapy
CBT	Cognitive behavioral treatment
CBT-BN	Cognitive Behavioral Therapy – Bulimia Nervosa
CFT	Conjoint family therapy
DBT	Dialectical behavioral therapy
EBT	Educational behavioral therapy
ED	Eating disorder
EDE	Eating Disorder Examination
EDNOS	Eating disorder not otherwise specified
EE	Expressed emotion
EOIT	Ego oriented individual therapy
FBT	Family based therapy
FPP	Focal psychoanalytic therapy
FT	Family therapy
GAF	Global assessment of functioning
HDRS	Hamilton Depressive Rating Scale
IPT	Interpersonal therapy
NICE	National Institute of Clinical Excellence
SFT	Separated family therapy
SPT	Self psychological therapy
SSCM	Specialist supportive clinical management
YBC-EDS	Yale-Brown-Cornell Eating Disorder Scale

Psychotherapies for EDs include both individual and, because current practice has incorporated an important role for the family in the recovery process, family therapies. The Maudsley family therapy for adolescents with AN who live at home with their parents has shown the best empiric outcomes.

In clinical practice, psychodynamic approaches represent an important component of the treatment for young people with EDs, although there are very few clinical research studies of individual or family psychodynamic therapy treatments of EDs. This article reviews the existing studies of psychodynamically informed therapies for the treatment of EDs. In general, the findings have been ambiguous, but they deserve further clarification, and, although limited, suggest that further research into psychodynamic treatments of EDs in youth is warranted.

Finally, we look at the gap between what is practiced and what is researched, concluding with recommendations regarding future directions for researching psychotherapy for vulnerable youth with EDs to better support clinicians in their efforts to treat the complex patients who present in the clinical setting.

BACKGROUND

Epidemiology of EDs in Youth

Case register studies depict the incidence rates for EDs in girls ages 10 to 14 to be between 25.7 and 26.3 per 100,000 and 3.3 and 3.7 per 100,000 for boys.[1–3] Both AN and BN show peak age of onset during adolescence.[4] AN first occurs at a younger age than BN.[5]

The prevalence of AN in 15-year-old to 19-year-old females is estimated to be between 0.48% and 0.70%. The prevalence of BN in the adolescent population is approximately 1% to 2%, whereas an additional 2% to 3% show clinically significant bulimic behaviors, but fall shy of the criteria for the full syndrome.[1–3] Thus, many, if not most young patients presenting for treatment would be classified as eating disorder not otherwise specified (EDNOS), a topic generally neglected in the research.[6,7] In comparison with case register studies, community studies for adolescent females show the lifetime prevalence to be 2.3% for AN or BN.

Compared with other psychiatric illnesses, EDs have high levels of mortality. The standardized mortality rate for AN (5.86 per 100,000) is 12 times higher than for the general population of females aged 15 to 24.[8] For BN the rate is 1.93.[9] The main medical complications for EDs are electrolyte disturbances, cardiovascular abnormalities, endocrine disorders, and osteopenia/osteoporosis, as well as gastrointestinal and hematologic complications.

Rarely do EDs present as the sole form of psychopathology, and individuals require a comprehensive psychiatric assessment to determine the presence of co-occurring disorders.[10,11] More than 50% of patients with an ED present with a mood disorder, most often, major depression. Over one-third of patients with an ED present with a co-occurring anxiety disorder, with obsessive compulsive disorder being the most prevalent. Treating the ED without treating the anxiety disorder, mood disorder, or substance abuse, makes the treatment of the eating disturbance virtually impossible. Similarly, to effectively treat the co-occurring disorders, it is critical to have nutritional rehabilitation. Furthermore, treating coexisting personality disorders, which may occur in up to 35% of patients with EDs,[12] is often necessary for recovery from the ED.

Understanding and treating EDs

Five decades after Hilde Bruch outlined a "modern" approach to working with children and adolescents with AN[13,14] and 3 decades after Gerald Russell described the syndrome of BN,[15] evidence-based treatments for children and adolescents with EDs remain a distant goal rather than a reality.

Bruch[13,14] understood that patients with AN were not suffering from loss of appetite, but that these youth were "frantically preoccupied with food and eating." She described their "relentless pursuit of thinness" as an outstanding symptom. She saw the ED as an effort to solve personality difficulties and problems of living. She also noted a "profound sense of ineffectiveness." For these patients, the AN was a way to measure self-worth. Turning to the role of the family, Bruch focused on the mother's behavior as either "responsive" or "stimulating," and the interaction with the child as "appropriate" or "inappropriate," depending on whether the mother's behavior fulfills the expressed needs of the child or disregards or distorts them.

Bruch[13,14] described her clinical work with adolescents with AN as derived from psychoanalysis with marked modifications of the classical psychoanalytic techniques, particularly rejecting deep interpretation and austere neutrality. She advocated establishing a collaborative atmosphere between therapist and patient. Bruch identified Harry Stack Sullivan as her most influential teacher. She also drew on the ideas of Heinz Kohut.

Russell coined the term BN for a syndrome of bingeing and purging he described as "an ominous variant of anorexia nervosa." He recognized the intensity of dysfunctional beliefs and distorted values concerning shape and weight, together with a "morbid fear of fatness," as the psychic underpinnings of BN and the driving force behind the subsequent loss of control of the bingeing and purging.

Based on Russell's descriptions[15] and CBT initially developed by Beck[16] and colleagues,[17] Fairburn and colleagues[18,19] developed and researched a CBT treatment approach: CBT-BN. CBT-BN focuses on change in the specific pathologic cognitions and beliefs and targets the cognitive disturbances overvaluing weight, shape, and appearance as determinants of self-worth, together with behavioral disturbances in weight and food regulation. CBT-BN aims to develop a regular pattern of eating, to reduce concern with weight, to cope with high-risk behaviors, particularly bingeing and purging, and to prevent relapse. CBT-BN, which involves 16 to 20 sessions over 4 to 5 months, is quite effective at eliminating binge eating and purging. CBT-BN added a new treatment pathway focused directly on the dysfunctional beliefs and values regarding shape and weight, which maintain the disorder. Russell[15] and Fairburn and colleagues[18,19] thought these beliefs needed direct attention in the treatment. CBT has been successfully adapted to the psychological treatment of EDs, especially BN and more modestly to AN. Of interest is our finding, as we reviewed psychotherapy research studies for this article, that positive outcomes did not necessarily require a focus on any of the symptoms of the ED.

A MULTIMODAL TREATMENT PLAN

Unlike many other psychiatric disorders (eg, depression) in children and adolescents, the treatment of youths with EDs involves a multidisciplinary team of providers whose work must be well-integrated to maintain its effectiveness. Additionally, the sequencing of treatments from across the biopsychosocial spectrum can affect the outcome. Teamwork can be undermined by the stress on clinicians of looming, life-threatening medical complications. For many patients, the ED symptoms are ego-syntonic, at the very core of the patient's sense of self, fueling resistance to the goals of the treatment, which must include weight gain and/or cessation of binge/purge cycles.

The multidisciplinary team may include, but is not limited to, physicians (pediatric and/or adolescent specialists), psychiatrists, psychologists, nutritionists, and social workers. In a hospital setting, the team may additionally include a nurse/nurse practitioner, child-life specialist, art/music therapist, and mental health worker. As in management of any illness, coordination between the professionals is crucial. The professional chosen to lead the team will depend on the clinical situation and particular characteristics of the individuals and the family involved.

Medical Evaluation and Re-feeding Come First

Before psychological interventions can begin, a full physical examination and laboratory studies including blood work, electrocardiogram, and any other studies that are clinically indicated (for example, electroencephalogram), must be completed to assess the patient's physical condition and identify possible medical complications from the ED. Re-feeding and weight gain are of ultimate importance. Without nutritional stabilization, progress in psychotherapy is limited and success elusive. Chaotic eating, bingeing, and vomiting need to be monitored and addressed. A starving brain, emaciated body, and out of control eating patterns disrupt the cognitive capacities, including attention and self-reflection, needed for psychotherapy to be effective.

The Psychotherapeutic Component of the Multimodal Treatment of EDs in Youths

Although there is no recovery from EDs without weight gain or cessation of the binge/purge cycle, change in these areas alone is not enough for a lasting recovery. For a sustained recovery, the psychological underpinnings of the disorder must be addressed. For patients with an ED, the sense of self in its many facets (eg, self-concept, self-esteem, self-control), developmental tasks, and interpersonal difficulties have become enmeshed in the distorting focus on weight. The goals of the psychotherapy are behavioral, social, and psychological. A change is sought in ED behaviors (restricting, binge eating, and self-induced vomiting), with a goal of establishing safe eating. Social treatment goals may include resolution of environmental stressors and cooperation within the family. Psychological treatment goals may include development of better coping skills and stabilization of comorbid psychiatric conditions. Longer-term psychological goals aim to resolve underlying vulnerabilities, such as a fragile self-esteem, negative self-image, and deficits in self-confidence, as well as to develop the ability to regulate affects without resorting to disordered eating behaviors or other self-destructive behaviors.

Methodology for This Review

This article reviews studies of psychodynamically informed therapies for the treatment of EDs that can contribute to the treatment approaches with children and adolescents. Our selection of studies for review required that the studies include some youth in their sample and include a psychotherapeutic treatment arm (whether the experimental cell or the control cell) that was deemed to be psychodynamically informed therapy as described in the next section. In addition, issues of good study design were considered by examining methodology, sample size, diagnoses of AN or BN based on the *Diagnostic and Statistical Manual of Mental Disorders* or *International Classification of Diseases*, and adequate descriptions of outcome using measures of weight gain, normalized eating, psychiatric diagnosis, psychological functioning, and physical health (**Table 1**).

Psychodynamically Informed Psychotherapies

Psychodynamically informed therapies draw on the rich tradition of psychoanalytic thought and psychodynamic psychotherapy techniques. Psychodynamic features we looked for when selecting studies to review included (1) focus in the therapy session on the subjective experience of the patient; (2) attention to the defensive operations by which the patient wards off painful thoughts and emotions; (3) appreciation for the interactions between the patient and the therapist, transference and countertransference, as a source of clinical information and as a therapeutic relationship; (4) focus on unconscious and psychodynamic meaning of symptoms within a developmental framework; and (5) awareness of patterns of past relationships and conflicts in present relationships. Some psychodynamically informed therapies are clearly derived from a school of analytic thought, such as ego psychology, object relations theory, or self-psychology, whereas others draw on the core concepts without referring to a specific school.

DESCRIPTIONS OF PSYCHODYNAMICALLY INFORMED THERAPY

In this section, we describe chronologically the psychodynamically informed therapy approaches to the treatment of EDs in youth and adults (as most of the therapies have been applied initially to adults). We first describe the individual and then family therapies.

Individual Therapies

Interpersonal therapy

Interpersonal therapy (IPT) is the leading empirically supported alternative to CBT for BN.[20] IPT was developed as a short-term, focal treatment designed to alleviate depression.[21] In IPT, the primary emphasis is placed on helping patients identify and modify interpersonal problems that may be contributing to their maladaptive eating behaviors.[22] We have classified IPT as psychodynamically informed on the basis of its conceptualization of the psychological problems of BN as difficulties in the individual's relationships with important others in their lives, an idea that is essentially derived from object relations theory. Unlike the agenda-led sessions of CBT, IPT sessions are patient-led (except at the very beginning) and unstructured. The IPT therapist is nondirective and there is no homework.

Table 1
Studies of psychodynamic psychotherapy and eating disorders

Authors	Subjects (No. Patients)/ Study	Study Location and Setting, Age	Diagnosis	Therapy	Measures	End of Treatment	Follow-up Evaluation/Assessment
Agras et al,[37] 2000	229	US: OP; mean: 28 (7) CBT: 28 (7) IPT: 28 (7)	BN; DSM-IIIR	CBT; IPT[a]	SCL-90-R, GSI, EDE, Inventory of Interpersonal Problems, SAS (self-report), RSES	CBT significantly superior to IPT in participants' recovery, remission, and eating attitudes and behaviors.	No significant differences between CBT and IPT by 12-month follow-up.
Bachar et al,[27] 1999	33	Israel: OP; mean BN: 24 (3) mean AN:18 (2)	BN, AN; DSM-IV	SPT[a]; COT; C/NC	DSM-SS; EAT26; BSI; SQ	SPT positive outcomes for AN and BN. COT nonspecific improvement. No changes detected after C/NC.	
Carter et al,[41] 2011	43	New Zealand: OP; age range: 17–40	AN; DSM-IV	CBT; IPT[a]; SSCM	GANM, EDE, EDI-2, GAF, HDRS		No significant differences on outcome measures between CBT, IPT, and SSCM at long-term follow-up (averaging 7 y). IPT more effective than SSCM at long-term follow-up. CBT remained stable over time.
Dare et al,[23] 2001	84	UK: OP; mean: 26 (7)	AN; DSM-IV	FPP[a]; FT[a]; CAT[a]; routine (control)	MR-Ave, BMI, ABW	At year 1, no statistically significant differences between groups on the MR rating scales Differences in weight gain in the specialized psychotherapies. FPP and FT significantly superior in weight gain compared with controls Most patients remained significantly malnourished.	

Eisler et al,[35] 1997	80	UK: OP; age range: 14–55	AN, BN; DSM-III-R	FT[a], Individual Supportive[a] (control)	ABW, MR-Scales		Significant improvements at 5-year follow-up found in the group, mainly owing to natural outcome of AN. FT favored with patients with EOSH-AN. Individual supportive therapy favored with patients with LO-AN.
Eisler et al,[34] 2000	40	UK: OP; age 16 (2); age range: 12–18	AN; DSM-IV or ICD-10	CFT[a], SFT[a]	SMFQ, RSES, MOCI, EAT, EDI, MR-Scale, BMI, FACES III, SCFI, EE	Significant gains in nutritional and psychological states with both groups Families with high EE, SFT better outcome than CFT. CFT had better on individual psychological functioning.	
Fairburn et al,[18] 1991	75	UK: OP; mean: 24; age range: 17 and older	BN; DSM-III-R	CBT, BT, IPT[a]	EDE-10, EAT, SCL-90, BDI, SAS (British adaptation)	All 3 treatments (CBT, BT, IPT) showed improvement on psychopathology. CBT more effective than IPT in attitudes to weight and shape, diet, and vomiting. CBT better than BT in modifying attitudes and dieting.	
Fairburn et al,[19] 1993	75	UK: OP; mean 24; age range:17 and older	BN; DSM-III-R	CBT, IPT[a], BT	EDE-10, EAT, SCL-90, BDI, RSES, SAS (British adaptation)		CBT and IPT equivalent and superior to BT at 12- mo follow-up. IPT took longer to achieve effects.

(*continued on next page*)

Table 1
(continued)

Authors	Subjects (No. Patients)/ Study	Study Location and Setting, Age	Diagnosis	Therapy	Measures	End of Treatment	Follow-up Evaluation/Assessment
Geist et al,[45] 2000	25	Canada: IP/OP FT mean 14 (2) FGP mean 15 (2) age range: 12–17	AN; DSM-IV (including <90% of IBW)	FT[a], FGP	DICA-R, EDI-2, CDI, BSI, FAM-III	FT and FGP significant weight restoration during the 4-month period. No significant changes in psychological functioning in FT and FGP.	
Lock et al,[33] 2005	86	US: OP long-term: mean 15 (2) short-term: mean 15 (2) age range: 12–18	AN; DSM-IV	FBT[a]	EDE, SADS-SAC, YBC-ED, CBCL, YSR, FES, BMI	Short-term FBT as effective as long-term FBT. Long-term FBT better for eating-related obsessive compulsive thinking and nonintact families.	
Lock et al,[30] 2010	121	US: OP AFT: mean 15 (2) FBT: mean 14 (2) age range: 12–18	AN; DSM-IV	FBT[a], AFT[a]	EDE, IBW, BMI, SADS-SAC	No differences in full remission rates. FBT superior to AFT for partial remission, improvement in BMI, and changes in the EDE.	FBT superior to AFT in full remission rates at 6- and 12-mo follow-up. No differences between groups in rates of partial remission, improvement with BMI, and changes with the EDE at 1- y follow-up.
McIntosh et al,[39] 2005	56	New Zealand: OP age range: 17–40	AN; DSM – IV	CBT, IPT[a], SSCM	GANM, EDE, EDI-2, GAF, HDRS	SSCM superior to IPT and CBT on global anorexia nervosa measure. CBT intermediate in response on many secondary outcome measures. IPT least effective.	
Murphy et al,[40] 2005	21	UK: OP BN: mean 28 (7); age range: 17–42	BN, BED; DSM-IV	Time-limited; Integrated[a]	BMI; frequency of bulimic behaviors	Bulimic behaviors significantly improved during psychodynamic treatment in BN. BMI relatively the same.	For BN, BMI remained unchanged. Improvement of bulimic behaviors maintained at 3- and 6-mo follow-up.

Robin et al,[43] 1994	22	US: OP BFST: mean 15 (3) EOIT: mean 14 (2); age range: 12–19	AN; DSM-IIIR	BFST, EOIT[a]	BMI, EAT, BSQ, Ineffectiveness, Interpersonal Distrust, and Interoceptive Awareness Scales of the EDI, BD , PARQ	BFST and EOIT improved significantly on BMI, although BFST produced greater gains than EOIT. Both treatments produced improvement on eating attitudes, body shape dissatisfaction, interoceptive awareness, depression/internalizing psychopathology, and eating-related family conflict.	
Robin et al,[29] 1995	22	US: OP BFST: mean 15 (3) EOIT: mean 14 (2) age range: 12–19	AN; DSM-III F.	BFST, EOIT[a]	BMI, PARQ, IBC	BFST and EOIT positively impacted BMI, menstruation, and family interaction. Mothers reported improvements in positive communication with BFST. Both groups had substantial reductions in negative communication and parent-adolescent conflict.	BMI, menstruation, family interaction, and improvements in eating-related conflict positively maintained 1 y following treatment.
Robin et al,[44] 1999	37	US: OP Age range: 11–20	AN: DSM-III R	BFST, EOIT[a]	BMI, EAT, EDI, BDI, CBCL, PARQ	BFST and EOIT effective treatments for AN. BFST had improved weight gain and resumption of menses.	Treatment gains maintained on all variables with both groups. By 1-year follow-up no significant differences between groups regarding menstruation.

(*continued on next page*)

Table 1
(*continued*)

Authors	Subjects (No. Patients)/ Study	Study Location and Setting, Age	Diagnosis	Therapy	Measures	End of Treatment	Follow-up Evaluation/Assessment
Russell et al,[42] 1987	80	UK: IP/OP mean 22 (7)	AN; BN DSM-III	FT[a], IT (supportive)[a]	MR-scale (AN), MR-scale (modified BN); ABW; CCEI	FT more effective than IT for patients whose illness began before 19 years of age and was not chronic. IT more effective than FT in patients whose illness begins at a later age.	
Treasure et al,[25] 1995	30	UK: OP EBT: mean 25 (7) age range: 18–39 CAT: mean 25 (5) age range: 18–35	AN; BN ICD-10	EBT, CAT[a]	MR-scales, ABW, BMI	After 1 year, both CAT and EBT had improvements with weight gain. Self-reported improvements higher with CAT than EBT. Severity of weight loss only predictor of outcome. Participants with greater weight loss had poorer response to treatment.	

Abbreviations: ABW, average body weight; AFT, adolescent-focused therapy[a]; AN, anorexia nervosa; BDI, Beck Depression Inventory; BE, binge eating; BED, binge-eating disorder; BFST, behavioral family systems therapy; BMI, body mass index; BN, bulimia nervosa; BSQ, Body Shape Questionnaire; BSI, Brief Symptom Inventory; BT, behavioral therapy; BSI, Brief Symptom Inventory; C, controlled; CAT, cognitive-analytical psychotherapy[a]; CBCL, Child Behavior Child Checklist; CBT, cognitive-behavioral therapy; CCEI, Crown Crisp Experiential Index; CDI, Children's Depression Inventory; CFT, conjoint family therapy[a]; C/NC, control/nutritional counseling; COT, cognitive orientation treatment; DICA-R, Diagnostic Interview for Children and Adolescents-Revised; DSM-SS, DSM Symptomatology Scale for Anorexia and Bulimia; DSM-IIIR, Diagnostic and Statistical Manual of Mental Disorders, third edition revised; DSM-IV, Diagnostic and Statistical Manual of Mental Disorders, fourth edition; EAT, Eating Attitudes Test; EAT26, Eating Attitudes Test 26; EBT, educational behavioral therapy; ED, eating disorder; EDE, Eating Disorder Examination; EDE-10, Eating Disorder Examination (10th Revision); EDI, Eating Disorder Inventory; EE, expressed emotion; EOIT, ego-oriented individual therapy[a]; EOSH, early onset and short history; FACES III, Family Adaptability and Cohesion Evaluation Scales; FAM III, Family Assessment Measure; FBT, family-based therapy[a]; FGP, family group psychoeducation; FES, Family Environment Scale; FKB-20, German Language Body Image Questionnaire; FPP, focal psychoanalytic psychotherapy[a]; FT, family therapy[a]; GAF, Global Assessment of Functioning; GANM, Global Anorexia Nervosa Measure; GCBT, group cognitive behavioral therapy; GPIP, group psychodynamic interpersonal psychotherapy[a]; GR, group; GSI, Global Severity Index; HDRS, Hamilton Depression Rating Scale; IBW, ideal body weight; IBC, Interaction Behavior Code; ICD-10, International Classification of Diseases and Related Health Problems, 10th Edition; INDIV, individual; IPT, interpersonal psychotherapy[a]; IT, individual therapy; LIFE Eat II, Eating Disorders Longitudinal Interval Follow-up Evaluation; LO, late onset; M, meta-analysis; Mo, month; MOCI, Maudsley Obsessive Compulsive Index; MR, Morgan-Russell; MR-Ave, Morgan-Russell Average Score; MR–GO Cat, Morgan Russell General Outcome Categories; NR, not reported; OP, outpatient; PARQ, Parent Adolescent Relationship Questionnaire; PCB, physical, cognitive, and behavioral; PSR, Psychiatric Status Rating Scale for Anorexia Nervosa; R, randomized; RC, randomized controlled; RSES, Rosenberg Self- Esteem Scale; SADS-SAC, Schedule for Affective Disorders and Schizophrenia for School-Aged Children; SAS, Social Adjustment Scale; SCFI, Standardized Clinical Family Interview; SCL-90, Symptom Check List-90; SCL-90R, Symptom Check List 90-Revised; SFT, separated family therapy[a]; SMFQ, Short Mood and Feeling Questionnaire; SSCM, specialist supportive clinical management; SPT, self-psychological treatment[a]; SQ, Selves Questionnaire; YBC-ED, Yale-Brown-Cornell Eating Disorder Scale; YSR, Youth Self-Report.

[a] Psychodynamic therapeutic components.

Focal psychoanalytic therapy

Focal psychoanalytic therapy (FPP) involves a standardized, time-limited, psychoanalytic therapy for treatment of ED in which the therapist takes a nondirective stance.[23] The therapy derives from the focused, short-term psychoanalytic psychotherapy of Malan.[24] The therapist focuses on the conscious and unconscious meanings of the symptoms, the patient's current relationships, and transference issues.

Cognitive analytic therapy

Cognitive analytic therapy (CAT) builds on educational behavioral therapy (EBT), a therapy that involves educating participants about AN and creating a behavioral regimen to help them accomplish adequate weight gain. In EBT, participants are encouraged to discuss issues regarding weight, body shape, and the goal of weight gain. Information and education regarding AN, nutrition, and metabolism are given. CAT combines cognitive therapy and brief, focused, psychodynamic psychotherapy. CAT differs from EBT in that it incorporates psychodynamic factors and focuses on interpersonal and transference issues.[25] The patient and therapist create a written formulation of the history of the ED and current problems. CAT focuses on interpersonal relationships both in the treatment (transference) and in the patient's history and social environment.[23]

Self-psychological therapy

Self-psychological therapy (SPT) views EDs through the lens of self-psychology. In the ED condition, food becomes a self-object of preference as opposed to other self-needs. As the patients progress with treatment, they begin to regard humans as self-objects instead and the ED begins to resolve. SPT is based on Kohut's work[26] and thus is the only psychotherapy for EDs explicitly based on an existing, longstanding, eponymously named psychodynamic theoretical model.[27,28]

Ego-oriented individual therapy

Ego-oriented individual therapy (EOIT) involves helping adolescents understand their individual strengths, while recognizing interpersonal issues that are occurring at the same time. The therapist serves as a "tension regulator," helping adolescents cope better with their dysfunctional families and choose alternative methods to self-starvation to gain control of their lives. Families are invited to collateral sessions and learn ways to cope with their children.[29]

Adolescent-focused individual therapy

Adolescent-focused individual therapy (AFT), used as the control arm in Lock and colleagues'[30] study of family-based therapy, is a commonly used model of therapy for those suffering with AN. AFT involves a year-long course of weekly individual psychotherapy with the goals of enhancing autonomy, self-efficacy, individuation, and assertiveness. Adolescents learn to identify and tolerate negative emotions. As opposed to CBT, which emphasizes thoughts and emotions surrounding food, AFT takes a more psychodynamic focus on mental states and coping with challenges and stresses of adolescence.

AFT consists of 3 main phases. The first phase includes establishing a rapport with the adolescent patient, as well as developing a summary of issues leading to the ED. The second phase emphasizes individuation, and how conflicts over individuation pertain to peer relationships, school or work, and family. In the third phase, the adolescents begin to develop suitable coping strategies for their adolescent problems, including sex, drugs, school, and peer stressors. Treatment and intervention strategies are thus aimed to target issues surrounding independence, anger, control, depression, and lack of self-esteem.[31]

Family Therapies

Family-based therapy

Family-based therapy (FBT) was developed by Dare and colleagues[32] at the Maudsley Hospital in London specifically for the treatment of children and adolescents with EDs. Although family therapy has been used in the care of youth with AN since the 1970s, the Maudsley approach has emerged beginning in the 1990s. This family approach was based on the work of Malan,[24] who had pioneered the development of brief psychodynamic therapy. Malan focused on interpretation of unconscious processes and intrapsychic conflicts. Although the origins of this treatment make it one of the most clearly psychodynamically informed treatments, at its core is a behavioral re-feeding intervention that uses the family as a fundamental resource in the treatment of the ED symptoms. This differentiates it from previous family therapy models. Over the years, this family treatment has been called the Maudsley treatment and/or family therapy (FT) and/or FBT. In the United States, Lock and colleagues[30] manualized the Maudsley method and continued the research. Regardless of how different researchers or clinicians label the approach, it is essentially a therapy in which families become a valuable, helpful resource to adolescents struggling with ED. The families are not looked on as the cause of the ED, but rather become instrumental in helping the adolescents take control of their life situations.

FBT addresses the ED as a problem of family dynamics, such as control battles, enmeshment, and conflict between family members. The parents are encouraged to take an active role in determining what their child eats. FBT sees patients battling with AN as "incapacitated" by their ED.[33] Initially, the child is identified as regressed in his or her ability to manage food independently. But, as re-nourishment is accomplished through collaboration within the family and weight is restored, responsibility for weight maintenance is shifted to the child.[22] Throughout, FBT explores the behaviors and thoughts associated with AN.

FBT is staged in the following 3 phases.

1. In phase 1, the parents unite in an attempt to develop a consistent approach to re-feeding their child. The therapist helps to dispel the notion that the parents have caused the ED. Not only do many parents feel they are to blame but also many youth do blame their parents.
2. Phase 2 begins when the youth has gained adequate weight. The parents begin to feel that they are effective in managing the care of their child. Symptoms of AN, which may include difficulty eating at public events, school, or at parties, continue to be a focus in the therapy. When the patient achieves stable weight gain and improves in her or his struggles with eating, phase 3 begins.
3. In phase 3, the adolescent identifies additional psychosocial stressors and concerns. The adolescents work toward autonomy and setting up age-appropriate boundaries within their families.[33]

Separated family therapy and conjoint family therapy

Separated family therapy (SFT) and conjoint family therapy (CFT) are 2 similar therapies that are distinguished by whether the therapist meets together with the patient and the family or with each separately. In SFT, although the family therapist works directly with youth and parents, sessions are divided among the parents and the patient, and the therapist does not directly observe interaction between family members in the sessions. The therapist takes a supportive role toward the family and the patient is encouraged to speak about his or her ED and about confrontations with family members. The aim is to develop an alliance between the patient and therapist. In CFT, the therapist works with the whole family in joint sessions and observes the interactions between the family members directly. The parents are encouraged to take an active stance with re-feeding their child, and the adolescent is encouraged to take control of his or her life.[34,35] Although the structure of the therapy is different technically, the approach is essentially FBT.

REVIEW OF THE RESEARCH STUDIES OF PSYCHODYNAMICALLY INFORMED PSYCHOTHERAPY

Results of Individual Approaches

We look at the research studies in chronologic order, except when there has been a follow-up study with the same subjects or a replication of treatment method in other locations. We present those results one after the other for continuity and clarity.

CBT and IPT

Fairburn and colleagues[18,19] in the United Kingdom were investigating CBT for BN and used IPT and behavioral therapy as the control arms. They concluded that CBT and IPT were more effective than behavioral therapy, and in early studies found lasting changes in all outcome domains. At this time, there have been 2 major randomized control studies (RCTs) of CBT and IPT for BN. These included 75 patients in the first 2 studies done in Oxford, England,[19,36] and 220 in the second study done in the United States by Agras and colleagues.[37] Both showed solid results. Agras and colleagues[37] later concluded that CBT-BN was superior to IPT in remission of binge eating and purging, as well as in the percentage of patients who recovered from the ED; however, there were no differences between CBT and IPT at 1-year follow up. As can be seen in **Table 1**, Fairburn and colleagues'[18,19] subjects were a combination of youth and adults, whereas Agras and colleagues'[37] subjects were adults only.

In contrast to BN, there have been few controlled trials of individual psychotherapy for AN, probably owing to the complexity and severity of the disorder and its relatively low prevalence.[38] Initial studies of CBT for adults with AN have shown limited effectiveness except for individuals with weight-restored AN.

A review of the literature on psychodynamically informed psychotherapy for the adult population with EDs (ie, a mixture of subjects with AN or BN), found 4 RCTs.[23,25,27,39] Additionally, we found 1 pilot study using an integrative approach.[40] Looking at the findings and follow-up of these 4 studies, we see that most of the time the results for treatment approaches that include psychodynamic features are comparable to CBT.

CAT and EBT

In 1995, Treasure and colleagues[25] compared CAT with EBT in a randomized trial of 30 patients and showed positive results. After 1 year, both CAT and EBT showed improvement with weight gain. Self-reported improvements using the Morgan Russell (MR) rating scales were higher with CAT than EBT. Severity of weight loss appeared to be a significant predictor of outcome. Participants with greater weight loss had a poorer response to treatment.

Self-psychology treatment

In 1999, Bachar and colleagues[27] showed positive outcomes with SPT for AN and BN with a slightly younger cohort than most of the studies we reviewed, but a fairly small sample of 33 patients. The cognitive orientation therapy arm of the study showed small improvements that were not statistically significant. No changes were noted with the control/nutritional-counseling group.

Randomized therapy

In 2001, Dare and colleagues[23] compared 3 specific psychotherapies for adults with AN. In this trial, 84 subjects were randomized to 4 treatments (FPP, CAT, FT, and low contact "routine" treatment) for 1 year. The study used the MR interview to assess patients on domains of nutritional status, menstrual scale, mental state, psychosexual scale, and socioeconomic status. Body mass index (BMI) was also measured. At the end of treatment there were no statistically significant differences noted between the groups on the MR rating scales; however, there were differences in weight gain, favoring those in the specialized psychotherapies over the routine treatment control. Nevertheless, more than two-thirds of the patients remained abnormally underweight. FPP and FT were significantly superior in weight gain compared with the control group. CAT showed some benefit, although the difference from routine treatment did not reach clinical significance.

In 2005, McIntosh and colleagues[39] included IPT in a study of 3 different types of psychotherapy for women with AN (ages 17–40). In this trial, 56 women were assigned to 3 treatments: CBT, IPT, and specialist supportive clinical management (SSCM) as the control group. SSCM involved clinical management (ie, education, care, and support), as well as supportive psychotherapy. Each therapy included a manual-based treatment for a minimum of 20 weeks. The primary outcome was a global AN measure. Secondary measures included physical, cognitive, and ED measures. Tertiary measures included the global assessment of functioning (GAF) and Hamilton Depressive Rating Scale (HDRS). Thirty-five of the initial 56 women completed treatment. The results showed that those receiving SSCM had outcomes as good, if not better, than the active treatment on the global AN rating. For other measures, CBT was intermediary between IPT and the control. IPT was the least effective treatment of all.

In 2011, Carter and colleagues[41] conducted a long-term (averaging 7 years) assessment of McIntosh and colleagues'[39] study sample. Fifty-six women participated in the follow-up study. No significant differences on any of the outcome measures were found among CBT, IPT, and SSCM at long-term follow-up. Patterns of recovery with posttreatment and long-term follow-up were compared. Although SSCM was initially found to be better than IPT on the primary outcome measure at the end of treatment, IPT was found to have a better global outcome rating at long-term follow-up. Thus, as with the IPT treatment of BN, there appeared to be a "lag" effect for IPT. Participants who received CBT were described as having a "more stable course."

Results of Family Approaches

Russell and colleagues[42] conducted a clinical trial in 1987, involving 80 patients, some of whom were adolescents, with AN or BN. In this trial, patients received an early version of the Maudsley family therapy or individual supportive therapy. Family therapy was more effective in patients with nonchronic EDs and onset before age 19. Older patients did somewhat better with individual therapy. This individual therapy was "not a formal psychoanalytic psychotherapy" but rather was more supportive in nature.

Behavioral family systems therapy: ego-oriented individual therapy

In 1994, Robin and colleagues[43] studied 22 youth with AN, comparing behavioral family systems therapy (BFST) with ego-oriented individual therapy (EOIT). Both groups showed improvement in BMI, although BFST showed greater gains in this area by the end of treatment. Both groups showed improvements in other measures, including eating attitudes, body shape dissatisfaction, interoceptive awareness, depression and internalizing psychopathology, and eating-related family conflict. These gains were maintained at 1-year follow-up. Robin and colleagues[29] also studied the impact of these therapies on family conflict. BFST and EOIT both appeared to have significant reductions of family conflicts and negative communications. In 1999, Robin and colleagues[44] studied 37 adolescents with AN, and randomly assigned them to BFST or EOIT. Both groups improved in family attitudes, depression, and reduction of family conflict; however, BFST resulted in greater weight gain. BFST also had more rapid resumption of menstruation than EOIT at posttreatment; however, by the 1-year follow-up, the EOIT group had similar outcome.

Conjoint family therapy: separated family therapy

In 2000, Eisler and associates[34] compared conjoint family therapy (CFT) and separated family therapy (SFT), and showed that both groups had made considerable gains in nutritional and psychological states. For families with high expressed emotion, SFT had a greater overall, positive outcome than CFT. Symptomatic change was greater with SFT, whereas CFT had better gains on individual psychological functioning.

Family therapy: family group psycho-education

In 2000, Geist and colleagues[45] compared a brief treatment (4 months only) of family therapy and family group psycho-education (a less costly approach) and found no significant differences among a small sample of 25 adolescents who had been hospitalized with AN. Both groups had gained weight during this time.

Long-term family therapy: short-term family therapy

Lock and colleagues[30,33] conducted RCTs focusing exclusively on adolescents showing positive outcome for FBT. In 2005, long-term family therapy and short-term family therapy were compared. There were no differences on any of the outcome measures for those adolescents with most severe Yale-Brown-Cornell Eating Disorder Scale (YBC-EDS) symptoms; however, the long-term model was associated with higher BMI results in those with the most severe ED symptoms. The long-term treatment also showed better Eating Disorder Examination (EDE) results in those subjects with nonintact families.[33]

Adolescent-focused therapy: FBT

In 2010, Lock and colleagues[30] conducted one of the largest studies to date, involving a trial of 121 participants (ages 12–18) with AN. The subjects were randomized to adolescent-focused therapy (AFT) or FBT. The primary outcome measure was full remission (defined as greater than 95% expected weight for age, sex, and height) and mean global EDE score within 1 SD of community norms. Secondary outcome measures included partial remission (greater than 85% of expected weight for height including those in full remission) and positive changes in BMI (adjusted for age and sex), changes in the EDE score, and decreased eating-related psychopathology. Although there were no differences in full remission between treatments at the end of treatment, FBT was significantly superior to AFT on this measure at the 6-month and 12-month follow-up period. FBT was found to be superior to AFT for partial remission and improvement in BMI, as well as greater changes in the EDE score at the end of treatment; however, these improvements were not found on follow-up. In summary, although both groups had gains in full remission by the end of treatment, FBT appeared to have greater improvement during the follow-up period.

National Institute of Clinical Excellence Guidelines

As most of the psychotherapy research studies we examine in this article are international, we believe it is useful to bring an international perspective by looking at the

National Institute of Clinical Excellence (NICE) guidelines for grading evidence-based practices. NICE, which is a part of the National Health Service (for England and Wales), has developed evidence-based practice guidelines that have significantly affected clinical practice. Evidence supporting a recommendation is noted in grades. Grade A requires at least 1 RCT. Grade B includes well-conducted studies, but no randomized trials. Grade C is the lowest grade and clinical studies of good quality tend to be absent with this grade.[20]

NICE Grading for the Treatment of EDs

There are no BN studies in adolescents alone. The studies combined adolescents with adults, and in most of these, there is no indication of the number of subjects at particular ages. Especially with regard to BN, we are relying on studies of patients in early adulthood to later adulthood to guide treatment of children and adolescents. Although this is far from ideal, hopefully it provides reliable clues to elements of treatment that can be effective for all age groups.

As per NICE guidelines, CBT-BN has received a Grade A recommendation for treatment of adults with bulimia. CBT-BN has been more effective than antidepressants in bringing about complete cessation of bulimic behaviors, and appears to be the most effective form of psychotherapy for short-term use. Adolescents with BN may also be treated with CBT-BN adapted to suit their age, circumstances, and level of development, and including the family as appropriate. CBT-BN for adolescents received a Grade C. NICE guidelines give IPT a Grade B and recommend that it should be considered as an alternative to CBT-BN but patients should be informed that it could take as long as 8 to 12 months to achieve results. The NICE guidelines have rated most techniques for AN, both CBT and psychodynamically informed, with a Grade C. The exception to these disappointing findings is FBT for adolescents, which is designated as Grade B by the NICE guidelines.[20]

THE GAP BETWEEN RESEARCH AND PRACTICE

Although ED researchers strongly endorse cognitive-behavioral approaches to treatment, review of the literature suggests that many patients with EDs show limited improvement with cognitive behavioral approaches to therapy. Many clinicians use psychodynamic approaches in their work with individuals with an ED. Few researchers are testing these approaches.

Although RCTs are the gold standard for research in the era of evidence-based medicine, for clinical practice they are not necessarily the most useful gauge of what will work. One possible reason for this is that the research subjects are selected on narrow diagnostic criteria without complicating comorbidities. It is not unusual for individuals with EDs to have comorbid anxiety, depression, substance abuse, or personality disorders.[11] Thus, the typical patient seen clinically is often not the patient seen in the research studies.

Often, the time-limited, symptom-focused approaches, such as CBT, are less successful with more complicated patients, especially adolescents with personality pathology, who may be more treatment resistant and require longer-term psychodynamic approaches.[46] Clinicians desiring to practice evidence-based medicine are faced with the dilemma that despite the clinical interest in psychodynamic treatments, there are remarkably few controlled studies for psychodynamic approaches for EDs. Comorbidity, which can interfere with the effectiveness of CBT, plays an important role in clinicians' minds justifying the use of psychodynamic treatment with patients with an ED, particularly when a personality disorder is co-occurring. To date, use of dialectical behavioral therapy (DBT), an empirically tested treatment for personality disorders in suicidal women,[47] has been effectively researched for the treatment of adult EDs.[48] However, other successful personality disorder treatments, such as transference-based psychotherapy[49,50] or mentalization-based therapy,[51] have not yet been studied for use with patients with an ED.

There is a wide gap between research and practice in the clinical community, as most practitioners do not follow CBT for BN.[52] One bridge over this gap between researchers and clinicians is proposed by Tobin.[53] He describes combining cognitive-behavioral and psychodynamic approaches, a treatment he describes as a "coping strategies therapy." In this model, Tobin[53] remarks that the shorter the treatment, the more likely it is to resemble a behavioral approach. Conversely, the longer the treatment, the more likely it is to resemble a psychodynamic approach.

Thompson-Brenner and colleagues[54] examined the treatment of EDs occurring in the community practice of experienced professionals. About one-third of the treatments were identified as psychodynamic, about a third as CBT, and a third as integrative/eclectic. This same study identified overlap, integration, and use of eclecticism for most therapists working outside of university/research treatment centers. Other investigations indicate similarly wide usage of psychodynamic approaches in addition to CBT, especially as most treatments continue longer than the 12 to 20 weeks typically found in research protocols.

Thompson-Brenner and colleagues[54] reported that although clinicians treating individuals with EDs identified themselves as either psychodynamic or behavioral in orientation, both were using psychodynamic and behavioral treatments. CBT clinicians were more likely to engage in psychodynamic approaches when the patients had co-occurring personality disorders. Mussell and colleagues[55] also found that many therapists, who reported using CBT as their primary technique for EDs, were later surveyed and identified to be using techniques other than CBT or IPT as their primary theoretical approach.

Tobin and colleagues[56] surveyed 265 clinicians online and at regional and international ED meetings. They reported that virtually all clinicians who attend ED meetings were using psychodynamic approaches with their patients with an ED, regardless of how they described their theoretical orientation. In addition, combination treatments are commonly implemented. The findings of this study suggest that most clinicians use a wide array of ED treatment interventions drawn from empirically supported treatments, such as CBT-BN, and from other treatments that have no randomized clinical trial support. Despite concerns, there is no evidence that combining CBT with other modalities reduces the effectiveness of CBT.[22,57]

SUMMARY

Recent trials have supported the use of FBT for treatment of adolescents with AN. CBT remains the primary recommended treatment for adults with BN; however, there is also a role for other therapies, such as IPT. Psychodynamically informed therapies represent an important treatment option for young people with an ED, but research evidence remains limited in this area. Although psychodynamic principles and treatment are frequently incorporated into the care of children and adolescents with an ED, further prospective research will need to be conducted to clarify the most effective treatment and to determine what works, for whom and how or why the treatment works.

Recommendations for Future Research

Some evidence-based research has been translated into guidelines and manualized approaches and for some therapists, this amplifies the scientific status of their clinical interventions with patients; at the same time, for other therapists, a need for experience-based practices may feel less programmed, less constrictive, and more responsive to the individual patient. This research-practice gap notwithstanding, we do have suggestions for future research. To connect real-world patients with subjects in studies, those with EDNOS need to be included in the various protocols, as well as individuals with co-occurring personality disorders. It is also clear that further research must focus on applying available adult treatments to children and adolescents, while focusing on and elucidating necessary developmental modifications and on integrative therapies combining elements of CBT and psychodynamic therapy. Regarding FBT, it would be helpful to also include an individual treatment for the adolescent, as this may enhance the benefits of working with the whole family. Little has been written about whether siblings need to be included in the family work and this may provide an interesting future focus. EDs are complex and challenging and not amenable to simple "do's" and "don'ts," but require integrating the best knowledge currently available together with clinical expertise. The clinical challenge that remains is how to match the most effective treatment to each patient and family to optimize recovery from these serious disorders.

REFERENCES

1. Hoek H, Hoeken DV. Review of prevalence and in incidence of eating disorders. Int J Eat Disord 2003;34(4):383–96.
2. Lucas AR, Crowson C, O'Fallon WM, et al. The ups and downs of AN. Int J Eat Disord 1999;26(4):397–405.
3. Pawluck D, Gorey K. Secular trends in the incidence of AN: integrative review of population-based studies. Int J Eat Disord 1998;23(4):347–52.
4. Mitchell J, Seim HC, Colon E, et al. Medical complications and medical management of bulimia. Ann Intern Med 1987;107(1):71–7.
5. Madden S. Evidence-informed care of children with eating disorders. In: Dancyger IF, Fornari VM, editors. Evidence based treatment for eating disorders: children, adolescents, and adults. New York: Nova Science Publishers; 2009. p. 137–54.
6. Fisher M. Medical and nutritional treatment of children, adolescents, and young adults with eating disorders. In: Dancyger IF, Fornari VM, editors. Evidence based treatment for eating disorders: children, adolescents and adults. New York: Nova Science Publishers; 2009. p. 119–35.
7. Peebles R, Wilson JL, Lock JD. How do children with eating disorders differ from adolescents with eating disorders at initial evaluation? J Adolesc Health 2006; 39(6):800–5.
8. Sullivan PE. Mortality in anorexia nervosa. Am J Psychiatry 1995;152:1073–4.
9. Arcelus J, Mitchell A, Wales J, et al. Mortality rates in patients with anorexia nervosa and other eating disorders: a meta-analysis of 36 studies. Arch Gen Psychiatry 2011;68(7):724–31.
10. Brewerton TD. Comorbid anxiety and depression and the role of trauma in children and adolescents with eating disorders. In: Jaffa T, McDermott B, editors. Eating disorders in children and adolescents. Cambridge (United Kingdom): Cambridge Univ Press; 2007. p. 158–68.
11. Fornari V, Kaplan M, Sandberg D, et al. The relationship between depression & anxiety disorders in AN & BN. Int J Eat Disord 1992;12:21–9.
12. Sansone RA, Levitt JL, Sansone LA. The prevalence of personality disorders among those with eating disorders. Eat Disord 2005;13(1):7–21.

13. Bruch H. Anorexia nervosa and its differential diagnosis. J Nerv Ment Dis 1966; 141:555–66.
14. Bruch H. The golden cage. The enigma of anorexia nervosa. Cambridge (MA): Harvard University Press; 1978.
15. Russell GF. Bulimia nervosa: an ominous variant of anorexia nervosa. Psychol Med 1979;9:429–48.
16. Beck AT. Cognitive therapy and the emotional disorders. New York: International Universities Press; 1976.
17. Beck AT, Rush AJ, Shaw BF, et al. Cognitive therapy of depression. New York: The Guilford Press; 1979.
18. Fairburn CG, Jones R, Peveler RC, et al. Three psychological treatments for bulimia nervosa. Arch Gen Psychiatry 1991;48(5):463–9.
19. Fairburn CG, Jones R, Peveler RC, et al. Longer-term effects of interpersonal psychotherapy, behavior therapy, and cognitive behavior therapy. Arch Gen Psychiatry 1993;50(6):419–28.
20. National Institute for Clinical Excellence. Eating disorders—core interventions in the treatment and management of anorexia nervosa, bulimia nervosa, and related eating disorders. NICE Clin Guideline No. 9. London: NICE; 2004. Available at: http://www.nice.org.uk/. Accessed May 2012.
21. Klerman G, Weissman M, Rounseville B, et al. Interpersonal psychotherapy of depression. New York: Basic Books; 1984.
22. Wilson GT. Psychological treatments of eating disorders. Annu Rev Clin Psychol 2005;1(1):439–65.
23. Dare C, Eisler I, Russell G, et al. Psychological therapies for adults with anorexia nervosa: randomized controlled trial of out-patient treatments. Br J Psychiatry 2001;178(3):216–21.
24. Malan DH. Toward the validation of dynamic psychotherapy. New York: Plenum; 1976.
25. Treasure J, Todd G, Brolly M, et al. A pilot study of a randomized trial of cognitive analytical therapy versus educational behavioral therapy for adult anorexia nervosa. Behav Res Ther 1995;33(4):363–7.
26. Kohut H. The Analysis of the Self. New York: International Universities Press; 1971.
27. Bachar E, Latzer Y, Kreitler S, et al. Empirical comparison of two psychological therapies. J Psychother Pract Res 1999;8(2):115–28.
28. DeGroot J, Rodin G. Coming alive: the psychotherapeutic treatment of patients with eating disorders. Can J Psychiatry 1998;43:359–66.
29. Robin AL, Siegel PT, Moye A. Family versus individual therapy for anorexia: impact on family conflict. Int J Eat Disord 1995;17(4):313–22.
30. Lock J, Le Grange D, Agras S, et al. Randomized clinical trial comparing family-based treatment with adolescent-focused individual therapy for adolescents with anorexia nervosa. Arch Gen Psychiatry 2010;67(10):1025–32.
31. Fitzpatrick K, Moya A, Hostee R, et al. Adolescent focused therapy for adolescent anorexia nervosa. J Contemp Psychother 2009;40(1):31–9.
32. Dare C, Eisler I. Family therapy for anorexia nervosa. In: Garner DM, Garfinkel P, editors. Handbook of Treatment for Eating Disorders. New York: Guilford Press; 1997. p. 307–24.
33. Lock J, Agras WS, Bryson S, et al. A comparison of short and long term family therapy for adolescent anorexia nervosa. J Am Acad Child Adolesc Psychiatry 2005;44(7):632–9.
34. Eisler I, Dare C, Hodes M, et al. Family therapy for adolescent anorexia nervosa: the results of a controlled comparison of two family interventions. J Child Psychol Psychiatry 2000;41(6):727–36.

35. Eisler I, Dare C, Russell G, et al. Family and individual therapy in anorexia nervosa: a 5 year follow-up. Arch Gen Psychiatry 1997;54(11):1025–30.
36. Fairburn C, Norman P, Welch S, et al. A prospective study of outcome in bulimia nervosa and the long-term effects of three psychological treatments. Arch Gen Psychiatry 1995;52:304–12.
37. Agras WS, Walsh T, Fairburn CG, et al. A multicenter comparison of cognitive-behavioral therapy and interpersonal psychotherapy for bulimia nervosa. Arch Gen Psychiatry 2000;57(5):459–66.
38. Bulik CM, Berkman ND, Brownley KA, et al. Anorexia nervosa treatment: a systematic review of randomized controlled trials. Int J Eat Disord 2007;40(4):310–20.
39. McIntosh VV, Jordan J, Carter FA, et al. Three psychotherapies for anorexia nervosa: a randomized, controlled trial. Am J Psychiatry 2005;162(4):741–7.
40. Murphy S, Russell L, Waller G. Integrated psychodynamic psychotherapy for bulimia nervosa and binge eating disorder: theory, practice, and preliminary findings. Eur Eat Disord Rev 2005;13(6):383–91.
41. Carter FA, Jordan J, McIntosh VV, et al. The long-term efficacy of three psychotherapies for anorexia nervosa: a randomized, controlled trial. Int J Eat Disord 2011;44(7):647–54.
42. Russell GF, Szumukler GI, Dare C, et al. An evaluation of family therapy in anorexia nervosa and bulimia nervosa. Arch Gen Psychiatry 1987;44(12):1047–56.
43. Robin AL, Siegel PT, Koepke T, et al. Family therapy versus individual therapy for adolescent females with anorexia nervosa. J Dev Behav Pediatr 1994;15(2):111–6.
44. Robin AL, Siegel PT, Moye A, et al. A controlled comparison of family versus individual therapy for adolescents with anorexia nervosa. J Am Acad Child Adolesc Psychiatry 1999;38(12):1482–9.
45. Geist R, Heinmaa M, Stephens D, et al. Comparison of family therapy and family group psychoeducation in adolescents with anorexia nervosa. Can J Psychiatry 2000;45(2):173–8.
46. Thompson-Brenner H, Weingeroff J, Westen D. Empirical support for psychodynamic psychotherapy for eating disorders. In: Levy RA, Ablon JS, editors. Handbook of evidence-based psychodynamic psychotherapy. New York: Humana Press; 2009. p. 67–92.
47. Linehan M. Cognitive-behavioral treatment of borderline personality disorder. New York: The Guilford Press; 1993.
48. Wisniewski L, Bhatnagar K, Warren M. Using dialectical behavior therapy for the treatment of eating disorders: a model for DBT enhanced CBT. In: Dancyger IF, Fornari VM, editors. Evidence based treatment for eating disorders: children, adolescents and adults. New York: Nova Science Publishers; 2009. p. 275–90.
49. Kernberg OF, Yeomans FE, Clarkin JF, et al. Transference focused psychotherapy: overview and update. Int J Psychoanal 2008;89:601–20.
50. Yeomans FE, Clarkin JF, Kernberg OF. A primer of transference focused psychotherapy for the borderline patient. Northvale (NJ): Jason Aronson; 2002.
51. Bateman A, Fonagy P. Psychotherapy for borderline personality disorder: mentalization based treatment. Oxford (United Kingdom): Oxford University Press; 2004.
52. Banker JD, Klump KL. Research and clinical practice: a dynamic tension in the eating disorder field. In: Dancyger IF, Fornari VM, editors. Evidence based treatment for eating disorders: children, adolescents and adults. New York: Nova Science Publishers; 2009. p. 71–86.

53. Tobin DL. The rationale for psychodynamic psychotherapy in eating disorders. In: Latzer Y, Stein D, editors. Treatment and recovery of eating disorders. New York: Nova Science Publishers Inc; 2011. p. 1–11.
54. Thompson-Brenner H, Glass S, Westen D. A multidimensional meta-analysis of psychotherapy for bulimia nervosa. Clin Psychol Sci-Pr 2003;10(3):269–87.
55. Mussell MP, Crosby RD, Crow SJ, et al. Utilization of empirically supported psychotherapy treatments for individuals with eating disorders: a survey of psychologists. Int J Eat Disord 2000;27(2):230–7.
56. Tobin DL, Banker JD, Weisberg L. I know what you did last summer (and it was not CBT): a factor analytic model of international psychotherapeutic practice in the eating disorders. Int J Eat Disord 2007;40(8):754–7.
57. Waller G. Evidence-based treatment and therapist drift. Behav Res Ther 2009;47: 119–27.

Psychodynamic Approaches to Medically Ill Children and Their Traumatically Stressed Parents

Ariane Schwab, MD[a], Sandra Rusconi-Serpa, PhD[b],
Daniel S. Schechter, MD[a,*]

KEYWORDS

- Chronic illness • Trauma • Parental PTSD • Psychodynamic psychotherapy
- Mentalization • Pediatric solid organ transplant • Consult-liaison psychiatry

KEY POINTS

- Psychodynamic thinking during the evaluation and intervention with chronically ill patients and their traumatically stressed parents can be both life saving and permit further emotional growth.
- Identifying risk versus resilience in the face of life-endangering illness is not so much dependent on the fact that patients and their families have experienced traumatic life events but rather, the meaning that is made of them within developmental and relational contexts.
- Efforts focus on understanding with children and families their psychological reactions to what is going on in the ill child's body, and inversely, the child's body's reactions to what is going on in the mind.
- Sensitively evaluating and treating traumatic stress among parents can render those parents more psychologically available to soothe their medically ill children.
- An important marker of positive change over the course of the consultation is improvement in coherence and richness of parent and child narratives about the child's experience and understanding of his or her illness and related interventions.

THE CONTEXT OF THE PEDIATRIC MENTAL HEALTH CONSULTANT

As consult-liaison psychiatrists and psychologists in a large university-based pediatrics hospital, we work within a multidisciplinary team caring for infants, children,

[a] Pediatric Consult-Liaison Unit, Child and Adolescent Psychiatry Service (SPEA), University of Geneva Hospitals and Faculty of Medicine, 51 Boulevard de la Cluse, 1205 Geneva, Switzerland; [b] Research Unit, Child and Adolescent Psychiatry Service (SPEA), University of Geneva Hospitals and Faculty of Medicine, 2 Rue Verte, 1205 Geneva, Switzerland
* Corresponding author.
E-mail address: Daniel.Schechter@hcuge.ch

Child Adolesc Psychiatric Clin N Am 22 (2013) 119–139
http://dx.doi.org/10.1016/j.chc.2012.08.007 **childpsych.theclinics.com**
1056-4993/13/$ – see front matter

adolescents, and their families. Our efforts center around understanding with children and families their psychological reactions to what is going on in the ill child's body, and inversely, the child's body's reactions to what is going on in the mind. The goal is to facilitate the best possible medical-surgical outcomes, psychological adaptation, ongoing development, and social-emotional support. As the children are the primary patients of the pediatricians and surgeons, we psychiatrists and psychologists remain as specialist-consultants. Thus, we do not decide on the larger frame of treatment as one might in a consulting room. We do not determine when the patients are admitted or discharged, although we can occasionally influence. Although we make suggestions, we do not write medical orders or prescriptions. We must work around an often unpredictable set of constraints set by the constellation of the patients' particular condition, hospital ward location, and scheduling of tests and medical-surgical interventions.

Nevertheless, as best we can, we intervene directly from the moment at which we are asked to consult. We place a premium on play with developmentally appropriate materials, including medical kits, ambulances, and hospital room scenes with human and animal figures. We also rely heavily on drawing, modeling clay, jointly attending with the patients to their interests in music, iPads (Apple Inc, Cupertino, California) and laptops, books, and manga at the bedside. As psychodynamically trained consultants, we take into account our multisensory observations, including our own emotional reactions and associations to our interactions with our patients and their families.

Our observations and reflections extend beyond those pertaining to patients and their families directly. As "an observing third",[1] we often address the interactions of the patient-family system with the medical-surgical team and nursing staff.[1] In a medical model that is increasingly subspecialized, our first priority becomes holding in mind patients as more than their disease or surgical procedure. We view who some refer to as *the liver transplant patient in room 109* as an individual child who has liver disease; is awaiting transplant; has particular somatic, psychic, social, and developmental context; and has a specific family and life history. In doing so, we can facilitate communication between patients and families as well as between them and the medical-surgical teams and consider countertransference elements that emerge among these health professionals involved in patients' daily care.

MENTALIZATION AS ONE IMPORTANT FOCUS OF ASSESSMENT AND INTERVENTION

Mentalization as described by Fonagy and colleagues[2] and as further developed by Slade and colleagues[3] is an important point of assessment and outcome in our work with ill children and their parents. Mentalization or *reflective functioning* as it is operationalized for purposes of measurement, is the person's capacity to think about what is going on in one's own mind as well as someone else's mind, both in terms of thoughts and feelings as well as to think about the interaction of their two minds. The capacity to hold in mind the mind of the other in relation to oneself is extremely important for mutual emotion regulation during early social-emotional development and eventual self-regulation of emotion.[4] In a study of violence-exposed traumatically stressed mothers and their young children, it became clear that the ability to mentalize is associated with the parent's having an integrated mental representation of their child and a relationship in which the parent is able to assist the child in his or her development of emotion regulation.[5] A caveat to this is that the more severe the maternal traumatization, the more likely that the mother will be compromised in her ability to exercise her mentalizing capacity, particularly at moments of interpersonal stress, such as separation, loss, and illness.[5,6]

Severe and chronic illness, particularly in children, arouses considerable conscious and unconscious reactions, foremost among them is anxiety among the parents and professionals taking care of them. As in the instance of violence-exposed traumatized parents and their young children, child chronic-illness exposed parents are also very often traumatized and have similar difficulties in their ability to exercise their capacity for needed mentalization, particularly when new medical challenges and stressors arise. This area is where our capacity to model and support the capacity to mentalize in others as psychodynamically trained mental health consultants who have had personal psychotherapy or psychoanalysis comes in very handy. As part of the medical community, our additional ability to offer feedback in language that is familiar to our non–mental health, medical-surgical colleagues with sensitivity to their particular contexts is invaluable.

LENSES THROUGH WHICH WE UNDERSTAND THE CHILD-PATIENT'S PERSPECTIVE

An essential aspect of psychodynamic work is its focus on individual patients who make meaning out of their own experience through the lens of all of their prior experiences. Particularly in the case of children, this lens is tinted and shaped by their developmental capacities and their relationships with caregivers and siblings. These developmental and relational contexts are crucial to understanding how illness affects the child emotionally.

Effects of Child Development

For infants and young children who are acquiring increasing mastery over bodily functions, illness and interventions can become embodied in such that they alter fundamentally their self-representation before the child's becoming verbal.[7] At any age, experiences—particularly traumatic ones, can create memory traces that are stored as bodily sensations and gestures. These traces are then said to be embodied.[7,8] Somatic memory traces from infancy and early childhood can, thus, be intensely visceral and lead the child to think that he or she had been born that way.

The psychodynamic technique in following patient affects and associations through verbal exchange, play, and nonverbal communication can render accessible embodied trauma even years after the most traumatic period associated with the illness. It is through the eyes of the parents as primary caregivers that the infant or young child identifies potential danger and makes sense of what is happening. As such embodied mentalization (ie, nonverbal caregiving behavior that is informed by parental mentalization and that takes into account the child's mind and bodily sensations) marks affective communication and rhythmicity in a containing manner and can help to attenuate the effects of embodied trauma.[9] So, when the parents' vision of the ill child is distorted or there is an impediment to taking the child's perspective and mentalizing, the mental health professional can serve a direct reparative role with the child as well as serving as a help to the parents.

Indeed, the health professional also becomes a caregiver to the child and family members. In an effort to keep the parents as protective caregivers, the medical team can become the source of alarm and danger rather than a source of help, support, and protection. Although the child's and family's transference plays a role here, as Viederman[10] describes, the reality of medical care easily reinforces patients' wariness. Enforced acceptance of the sick role at virtually all ages represents a threat, that is, a narcissistic injury to the individual's sense of invulnerability. Hospitals additionally tend to threaten narcissistic defenses and psychic integrity by bombarding patients with multiple encounters with a host of strangers who seem to have an intimate knowledge of the patients' body and vulnerability but no relationship with the patients. It is also invaluable to have a mental health consultant as an ally positioned between the patients and the medical staff. Thus, the priority of any consultation beyond ensuring the safety of the patients is the establishment and maintenance of the therapeutic alliance, which in turn is a potent predictor of the success of the intervention and ultimately compliance with the medical regimen.[11] The gradual co-construction of the child's, the parents', and their relationship's life narrative with the consult-liaison specialist can catalyze a powerful alliance as well as facilitate change in mental representations of self and other.[10]

Every developmental stage will have its particular challenges for the consult-liaison service. At about 7 years of age, as awareness of mortality and finality of death emerges, additional anxieties must often be addressed, including more profound feelings of guilt and remorse. The child who is chronically ill with frequent school absences and more or less visible constraints on his or her physical participation in social settings with peers can make children feel defective, marginal, isolated, and demoralized. They may have trouble keeping up with academic work. During adolescence, concerns about appearance, autonomy, competence in one's gender role, sense of future accomplishments, and romance create additional layers of worry. Compounding this is the possible effect of the chronic illness, related malnutrition, and treatments to stall the onset or progress of puberty such that adolescents feel out of synch with their peer group, more fragile, and stuck in the context of family, who may be stressed and unable to respond adequately to their needs.[12]

It is not surprising that severe chronic illness involving repeated hospitalizations and intensive-care-unit stays are associated with an increased prevalence of major depressive and posttraumatic stress disorders among children and adolescents—up to double the rate in the average population. The risk factors for these include premorbid psychiatric disturbances in the child and/or the parents, premorbid developmental difficulties, and the invasiveness of procedures.[13]

The Challenged Child-Parent and Family Attachment Relationships

Childhood is a time we like to imagine is joyful and carefree, far from death and disease. The suffering and dysfunction of the ill child, conferring a diagnosis, and scheduling interventions threaten the normative narcissistic defenses of parents and, in so doing, create a threat to their capacity to remain available to their child to assist in containing anxiety, regulating emotions, and representing a secure base. In this sense, the overwhelming or traumatic aspect of the illness, much as in the instance of interpersonal violence[5] can inhibit or attenuate the parent's normative capacity to mentalize, to think about what is going on in both the child and his or her own mind and body, feelings and thoughts, and to respond to the child's demands and questions with developmentally sensitive responses.

Importantly, as has been described in Schechter and colleagues's[14,15] work, the direction of effect is not exclusively from traumatized parent to child. The very young child, by virtue of his or her developmentally determined incapacity to regulate his or her own affect, distress, and aggression, exerts a powerful effect on the traumatized parent, such that the not-yet-traumatized child and the already-traumatized parent co-construct a new traumatogenic set of interactions, resulting in parental avoidance of the child's affective communication and in the child's increasing distress.

In the case of the medically ill child in a hospital setting, when a parent reacts by taking further distance, becoming overly permissive, or when the parent avoids visits with his or her child or misses important appointments with medical staff, not only is the child left more distressed but the parent will often seem to medical staff to be self-involved or otherwise insensitive to the child's needs as a bad parent rather than that the parent is trying to cope with an emotionally untenable situation. This situation can also occur if the parent becomes too overprotective and controlling at the expense of the child's emotional well-being. An essential part of our work is to address the mental health of the parent and the parent-child relationship following careful evaluation that includes systematic observation during individual parent interviews, parent-child (dyadic and triadic) visits, and family sessions.

A child's chronic illness can also place enormous additional stresses on the parental couple, with an increased risk of separation, financial instability, and difficulties for siblings whose parents are preoccupied with the ill child or depend on older siblings to help the parents at the siblings' expense. Severe family dysfunction and parental personality disorders can indeed be exacerbated by the threat of abandonment and family disintegration in the context of chronic illness and prolonged and repeated hospitalizations.[16]

MENTAL HEALTH RISKS TO PHYSICAL HEALTH

Emotional reactions to illness in children and their families can contribute to noncompliance with medical regimens critical to better outcomes and survival. There is already some evidence that psychodynamic approaches with chronically ill patients who have difficulty with medical compliance contribute to behavioral change, including greater medical compliance and greater insight in to their medical condition. Moran and colleagues,[11] for example, conducted a controlled trial of intensive psychoanalytic treatment of school-aged children who were unable to maintain a diabetic regimen (diet, injections, and exercise) and who consequently suffered from chronic dyscontrol of their blood glucose. Children in the psychoanalytic psychotherapy did significantly better in terms of blood glucose control than those who received only supportive consultation visits; there was also maintenance of better glucose control and indices of social-emotional development and understanding of their illness and their mental states 1 year later.

In the case of organ transplant, noncompliance can be fatal.[17] Nonadherence is the second highest cause of graft rejection in children and adolescents.[16] Shaw and colleagues[17] showed that for patients receiving renal transplants, nearly a third were noncompliant and that the strongest predictor was the presence of comorbid psychiatric illness in the child and/or one or both parents.

PRINCIPLES OF ASSESSMENT

When approaching chronically medically ill patients as psychodynamically minded consultants, we ask ourselves the following questions:

- What are the unstated, as well as the stated, motives of the consultation?
- How did the idea of consulting us come up? What was said?
- How do the child and parents understand why we are consulting? What are their expectations?
- Who lives with the child and how do they live?
- What are cultural, religious, and socio-economic factors that fit or do not fit with the child's context as presented?
- What external reality factors are adding stress and potentially constraining our capacity to intervene? Are there social issues and concrete needs (like housing) that put the therapeutic alliance in jeopardy?
- Who is/are the main attachment figures?

- What characterizes the important relationships in the child's life?
- What was the child's adaptation like before hospitalization?
- Where is the child in his or her development? What are his or her current needs and desires?
- What are the repercussions of the child's specific medical conditions and interventions on his or her current development and relationships?
- How might the child's emotional response and understanding of what is happening in his or her body and what will be done to his or her body be informed by his or her prior experiences, development, and relationships?
- What are the needs, wishes, and fears among different members of the family? How might these factors compliment or impede the needs of the child-patient being addressed by his or her parents, medical caregivers, and by us as mental health consultants?
- What are the needs, wishes, and fears among members of the multidisciplinary team that can help and/or hinder their care of the child?
- What transference, countertransference, versus real relationship elements come up during and even before the assessment and during the planning for our consultation?
- What is the reaction of the child and family members when we come in to see the child?
- Do the parents show an interest in exploring the emotional dimension of their child's and their own experience at the hospital?
- How much do the parents separate out their own emotional response and understanding of the child's experience from that of their child's?

SOURCE OF REFERRAL

In most instances, our consultation is requested by colleagues (physicians, social workers, nurses), which, from the beginning, introduces possible bias in the construction of the therapeutic alliance. Less often, patients and/or their families initiate the request. However, in certain circumstances, a psychiatric evaluation of patients and their families is formally required; and we are presented to patients and their families as just another part of the medical-surgical multidisciplinary team. This integration of mental and physical health from the point of initial assessment becomes an equalizer that overcomes much stigma that is often attached to requesting a mental health professional.

Such is the case of the pretransplant medical assessment; part of the protocol is for us to evaluate each patient considered for transplant, as well as that patient's family, before they can be placed on the waiting list for a donor organ. This practice allows for very useful preparatory work for accompanying families through an enormously stressful process that is filled with both hope and dread. When a transplant is successfully performed, patients and families face a new set of challenges to maintain the transplant, prevent potentially lethal rejections, and to deal with the side effects from the powerful immunosuppressive medications.

We will narrow our focus for the rest of this article on our work with patients and families seen in our hospital's liver transplant program.

CONSULTATION WORK WITH THE GENEVA LIVER TRANSPLANT CENTER

The Children's Hospital of the University of Geneva Hospitals is the Swiss national pediatric liver transplant center. Liver transplant is the only treatment option in cases of terminal liver failure as well as in 50% of cases of fulminant hepatitis.[18] All children in

Switzerland being considered for liver transplant, along with their caregivers, are seen by us before a transplant can take place. In the past 2 years, there have been an average of 7 transplants per year. Following a transplant in Geneva, these children are also followed up for their less specialized care in their own region's hospitals. The national versus regional continuity of care ends up requiring very complex collaboration, with multidisciplinary work requiring coordination across at least 2 different medical centers that are typically at some distance from one another.

Generally, patients enter the liver transplant program as infants and young children. The most common pediatric diagnosis associated with liver transplant is congenital biliary atresia. These patients enter our program very early, usually before 3 months of age. All of the patients receiving a liver transplant are generally followed at our hospital until 16 years of age, at which time they are transferred to the internal medicine department housed in the adult university hospital down the road. The frequency, duration, and composition of consultation visits (ie, patient alone, patient and family members) is variable depending on the condition, the wishes, and practical constraints specific to the situation of a given patient and their family.

In addition, because Switzerland has 3 national languages (German, French, and Italian) with additional immigrant families coming from all over the world, and with our national transplant center situated in the French-speaking region, we must often work with patients and their families in at least 2 languages, keeping in mind often very different cultural and socioeconomic backgrounds.

The following is a case example that illustrates how the psychodynamic approach to evaluation and subsequent intervention has helped to improve the medical and psychological outcome of a patient with a liver transplant receiving our services.

THE CASE OF PAUL AND HIS MOTHER ANGELICA

Paul, aged 10 years, suffers from Alagille syndrome, which includes severe cholestatic disease and renal insufficiency, and has been followed since early infancy by the gastroenterology clinic. Paul is an only child who resides with his mother Angelica in a small apartment in a remote German-speaking mountain village 5 to 6 hours away from Geneva by train. His mother has devoted her life to Paul's care. His parents have never lived together. His father was said to eat dinner with Paul regularly in his hometown, but was estranged from Paul's mother. He did not visit Geneva during Paul's hospital stay and remained avoidant of contact with the medical staff. The first author, Dr Schwab, was told before the evaluation that the medical specialists already foresaw huge problems collaborating with Paul. Indeed, the medication compliance was historically erratic, which worsened his physical health (progression of the liver disease) and adversely affected his appetite, food intake, and physical growth. The medical staff attributed this to his mother Angelica.

Paul speaks a Swiss-German dialect that is challenging for anyone who does not come from Paul's region. Even though speaking his language, pediatricians in their regional medical center reported a poor therapeutic alliance with the mother and 7 years of difficulty in following Paul because of irregular and unpredictable collaboration with Angelica that had resulted in a referral to child protective services.

There were several potential impediments to putting Paul on the transplant list. His pediatricians were afraid Angelica would completely block Paul's access to the treatment he needed to survive and was initially virulently opposed to the transplant. By the beginning of our intervention, this had turned to ambivalence. According to colleagues, the social services intervention did not help much, but Angelica seemed to understand that she had no choice and would have to keep coming to Geneva for Paul's medical follow-up. Our intervention led to reduced social service involvement, although there remained conflicts between the mother and the Geneva medical-surgical team as well as between the regional medical professionals and the Geneva team. Nevertheless, we saw hope and suggested a period of intervention before there was a final decision as to whether or not Paul would be on the transplant list. From a strictly medical point of view, Paul had met the criteria for transplant for years. But even with the significant worsening of his condition, the medical-surgical team would not put him on the transplant list because of the mistrustful and erratic nature of their relationship with his mother.

As often happens in cases of severe chronic illness, all the planning and measures of control falter if there is a turn for the worse. Indeed, Paul's condition worsened shortly after the decision was made to undergo a transplant, paradoxically leaving it as Paul's only viable option. It was at that point that the once muted message from the medical-surgical team became loud and clear: please change Paul's mother so that we can be reassured enough about a return on our efforts to transplant Paul—a tall order.

As psychodynamically trained consultants, we have the advantage of being trained to take our own psychic pulse before taking that of our patients (or their mothers). Even before meeting the patient, Dr Schwab felt confused, oscillating between hopelessness (there is no hope, even before trying), omnipotence (Dr Schwab thought maybe she would be the one who will succeed), and fortunately a combined sense of clinical curiosity and obligation to get to know Paul and his family and to be able to draw her own conclusions about why it was so hard for that mother to follow the medical advice. A very important part of the countertransference was the feeling of being annoyed with the medical-surgical team's being so judgmental. This annoyance became a potential source of connection to the mother; but if unmonitored, could lead to further splitting of good and bad part-object representations that could well complicate the coordination of care.

We began seeing Paul and Angelica for relatively brief 30-minute visits twice per week. See **Table 1** for the phases/stages of the therapeutic process, which took place over 1 year of the patient's hospitalization. The frequency and duration of visits increased over the first 3 months until Paul and Angelica were each being seen twice a week for 45 minutes, with an additional third joint mother-child session. Again, we present here the ideal frequency and duration of sessions (as discussed later); the practical reality often challenges this ideal such that we must adapt to working with the best possible treatment frame that can be realized.

Phase 1: Building a Therapeutic Alliance (Duration: 3 Months)

As soon as Dr Schwab entered the room, she was struck by the terrible sight of Paul's skin color, which had almost turned as green as the wicked witch of the West because

Table 1
Stages or phases of therapeutic process

In reviewing this therapeutic process itself, which took place over 1 year of hospitalization, the authors could divide it into 5 phases/stages:	
1. Building a therapeutic alliance	3 mo
2. Building tolerance for separation and anxiety	4 mo
3. Accepting the need for transplant, loss of the pretransplant life, and owning the desire for life posttransplant	~1 mo
4. Idealization of the transplant itself and of imagined life posttransplant	4 mo
5. Preparing to return home and transitioning to outpatient follow-up in the family's own region.	~3 mo

of his severe cholestasis. Her first thought was: *he looks so sick.* Paul was lying flat in the bed, avoiding eye contact, but then staring into his mother's eyes and only talking to her in their dialect, as if Dr Schwab did not exist. When she introduced herself to them, Angelica quipped with a sense of anxiety and annoyance that she does not need any help and neither does Paul. She said she had been seen by a psychologist for 3 years, who corroborated that everything is fine. Because Dr Schwab did not just leave but waited and took in what the mother was saying together with her own feelings of having been rejected and devalued, Angelica spontaneously added, "I'm not crazy," and then asked Dr Schwab curtly to leave the room. Although the first thought is to do as Angelica says, Dr Schwab waited and replied calmly, empathizing with Paul and his mother's terror, "I am not here because we think you or your son are crazy but because I am worried about Paul and you and how you are managing with this horrendously stressful situation." Angelica remained silent but was clearly listening, somewhat less tense but stone-faced. Dr Schwab told Paul and Angelica calmly and slowly that she would leave now but come back in a few days to see how Paul and Angelica were doing, adding while facing Paul, "because I think that being in the hospital must be really tough for you." Neither Paul nor his mother objected. During the following session, Angelica tolerated Dr Schwab's presence and used the whole session to explain how essential she is to her son's everyday life, how she is the only one who can care for him, knowing that she even makes the nurses feel useless. We hear for the first time that perhaps she feels useless, impotent in the face of Paul's illness, guilty, and desperate. Each time Dr Schwab spoke to Paul, he would not answer, or if she tried to talk about him to stimulate his participation, his mother immediately reacted in an overprotective and mistrustful manner: "But if you see him alone, what would you do with him?" Angelica clearly stated that she would accept or even encourage Dr Schwab to return but only if she were included in the sessions with the rationalization that, in that way, Paul would be more confident and comfortable using his own dialect. Dr Schwab reassured Angelica by following her lead, understanding and respecting her defensive, narcissistic posture by reinforcing that, as Paul's mother, she is essential to his treatment and even more, a true expert on her child. Angelica acquiesced to having regular consultation visits with reassurance that Dr Schwab would not separate Paul and his mother. The next stage would involve being able to make contact with Paul.

To allow for this, Dr Schwab suggested that the 3 play together. Because Paul and she had not played much at all during his many hospitalizations and because no other professional had tried this, Angelica seemed surprised but less threatened than by sitting up and talking. Mother's agreeing to play allowed Paul to choose his activity. Dr Schwab brought the basic kit of toys that includes a family doll set, a medical kit, an ambulance, aggressive and docile animals, play food and utensils, and drawing materials. Paul had a hard time deciding what he wanted to do. Hesitating, he looked at his mother; and seeing her nodding in approval while looking at the drawing materials, he chose to draw with markers. But again, he hesitated before choosing the color. He touched the red marker and looked up. Only once his mother had nodded a second time did he start to draw in red—a male character with a big sword. He wrote his name underneath it. Angelica encouraged him and clapped for the correct spelling of his name. Neither Paul nor his mother had once made eye contact with Dr Schwab. She felt as if she were not in the room until he finished his drawing. Only then, Paul smiled and, for the first time, lets Dr Schwab interact with him. She asked him what the boy/man was doing? He silently pointed out the sword. Dr Schwab continued after a pause, "he appears to me as a warrior, what's the fight about?" Paul seemed to ignore Dr Schwab but silently underlined his name. Because of the contrast between the submissive attitude of Paul and the vigorous opposition of the mother despite the severity of her son's disease, Dr Schwab, with a question in mind about how Paul might manage his aggressive impulses, intervened by saying, "Oh maybe this boy is you? Indeed, I can really well imagine how sometimes you might feel like fighting against the illness that makes your life so difficult! And I can imagine that you might also feel like fighting against the hospital itself..." He looked deeply into Dr Schwab's eyes, which was the first time he had not avoided her eye contact; but he remained silent. Angelica immediately interrupted the session and asked to speak alone with Dr Schwab. She said, "I don't want for you to talk to him about his disease, *he doesn't know*, I never told him, he is too young to hear about all that."

Dr Schwab was shocked. She wondered how it had been possible *not* to talk about Paul's disease? Dr Schwab told Angelica that she was very surprised about what Angelica had said and continued, "I understand that you want to protect your son—that's clear; but Madame, how do you explain to him his need for medications, procedures, even hospitalizations?" Angelica replied also in a surprised tone, "I don't...oh no, he never asks questions like that!"

This session was a critical turning point during this initial evaluation phase. Angelica and Paul were both draped in denial, a defensive armor implicitly shared by both. Angelica was clearly hostile. Each and every professional who entered the hospital room was perceived as a source of potential harm rather than help. And although not explicit, when Dr Schwab approached Paul, she felt as if she were a dangerous monster—a word that Paul would use much later to describe his fears when apart from his mother. We were tempted to interpret this mistrust and expectation of menace as a reaction to Paul's illness and the less-than-sensitive aspects of the hospital environment. However, Dr Schwab later learned that Angelica had a long history of profound mistrust of neighbors in her village and of the staff in Paul's school. She had blacklisted and filed formal complaints about several individuals, thus contributing to her reputation as being difficult.

Paul's mental state at that time was nearly impossible to evaluate. Angelica had essentially forbidden our asking questions of Paul and of Paul's curiosity about us, let alone about his condition, his hospitalization, or the rest of his life. Despite this, as Dr Schwab and our resident at the time gained Angelica's trust, they also began to ask Paul about his health, his wishes, and fears. They were met repeatedly with avoidance. Paul would change the subject or suddenly interrupt the session with the complaint of an acute pain or urgent need to drink or to go to the toilet. Even when not asked about issues that were emotionally charged, such as in efforts to engage in some free play, Paul had enormous difficulty in expressing his own interest or point of view. He typically would not initiate an activity but rather remain vigilant of his mother's every expression and gesture. When he received a sign of approval, he would choose a toy or activity as authorized nonverbally by his mother. This symbiotic functioning of mother and son, this interdependence with shared defenses of denial and avoidance suggested to us the likely fantasy shared by Angelica and Paul, namely, that as long as they would remain together, in league against all the others, nothing can happen to them. Any potential third in this dyadic system as Ogden described,[1] was viewed as a menace, hence, Dr Schwab's having felt as if she were a monster in the room.

As we built an alliance with Angelica, we began to learn more about her history that would explain how frightened and defended she was. Angelica was the last of 10 children and was born into a family of modest means. She described herself in relation to her siblings as an outlier who was perpetually in conflict with her sisters, whom she described as being jealous of her beauty. Angelica said that she always got along better with men than women, her brothers and father included. She identified her father as her primary attachment figure and described her mother as often distant and not looking out for her or being otherwise attentive to what was important to her when she was growing up. A particularly important backdrop to Angelica's experience with Paul is the fact that Angelica's father died of incurable liver cancer only a few years before Paul's birth. Angelica was devastated by his death. In tribute to her father, she chose to name Paul after her father whose passing she continued to mourn. Angelica's history, as she recounted it, was remarkable for descriptions of men who were either sick or otherwise dependent on women. Her brother remained single and living with her mother until she was placed in a nursing home at the age of 82 years, he was already 60 years old. The sum of these features of her history, including the fact that Paul reminded her of this favorite brother and her liver-diseased father, remained rather fixed determinant aspects of her mental representation of Paul and her relationship with him.

Angelica's adult history is characterized by her, for unclear reasons, never having completed her professional education, never having worked (before Paul was born when she was 42 years old), and her having lived on disability benefits for what she described as a syndrome of chronic fatigue and tendonitis. She described that she never had lasting romantic relationships with men because she was always betrayed or disappointed. As for Paul's father, she stated that they could never be together for more than a few months at a time because they would have repeated blowups. Her description of the relationship was extremely ambivalent and chaotic. When Angelica realized that she was pregnant, she was surprised and scared. When she found out the baby was a boy, she was relieved and hopeful. She denied any difficulty with Paul, despite her on-off relationship with Paul's father, until Paul's liver disease was diagnosed at 2 years of age.

This understanding of the mother and child psychic functioning allowed us to see the whole clinical case with different lenses:

1. There is significant psychopathology within the mother-child relationship that is characterized by psychological dissociation in the context of significant traumatization and the mother's disordered personality functioning (ie, with narcissistic; histrionic; and borderline features, such as profound mistrust and unpredictability, with prominence of psychological defenses such as splitting, devaluation and idealization in the context of her own history of trauma, loss, and troubled attachments This psychopathology must be addressed when working with the patient and his mother individually and together such that the clinician further evaluates and addresses the needs of each individual AND their relationship. For example, does Paul avoid asking questions or even formulating them so as to protect his mother's fragile ego in a role-reversed pattern? Or does Paul not think of any questions because he is in a submissive, regressed state? Will the mother remain rigid in her conviction that Paul has no curiosity about his condition? Will she be able to see, with help, her impact on the development and expression of his curiosity?
2. Our understanding of these issues must be translated into the succinct language that the medical-surgical team can take in. The effort must be directed to increase the multidisciplinary team's empathy for the child and mother via an emphasis on their being traumatized and frozen with fear so as to reduce the team's negative countertransference.

Once the emphasis was placed on the traumatic experience shared by Paul and his mother, and their distance perceived as avoidance caused by intense anxiety rather than defiance, all of the relationships changed: mother and Paul with each other but also mother and Paul with Dr Schwab and with the medical-surgical team and even Dr Schwab and the medical-surgical team. Why? Dr Schwab was, in a way described by the British psychoanalyst Wilfred Bion,[19,20] able to absorb the many unintegrated fragments, link them, which is to say link the mother's mental state and her behavior with her son's and their shared experience of a terrifying threat to Paul's body and life, and, by narcissistic extension, his mother and their relationship together. In other terms, Dr Schwab both modeled and stimulated mentalization for the patient, his mother, and the medical-surgical team.

This psychodynamic psychotherapeutic intervention permitted the mother to formulate and divulge additional traumatic factors that contributed to the observed psychopathology. At 3 years of age, Paul underwent 2 surgical interventions (one was a biliary derivation, related with the hepatic issue) and had a cardiac incident in the intensive care unit. In the mother's memory, this was a heart attack, a brush with death, and very traumatic. She recalled her helplessness and speechlessness as she saw her son dying in front of her. Following a second operation shortly thereafter, she was haunted by the sight of her son intubated and, this time, his speechlessness, which reminded her of the death of her mother following a stroke. Angelica and Paul remained in this speechless, questionless state such that Angelica could not even entertain the idea of a liver transplant, which revived images of cardiac arrest and intubation but not the idea of being a life-saving procedure for Paul. Indeed, the only experience Angelica had ever had of life-saving procedures was associated with the death of her first Paul, namely, her father who died despite the family's desperate efforts to keep him alive.

Another important aspect of the psychodynamic approach is the distinction between external and psychic reality. Although external reality in the face of illness is essential to validate as much as possible, the relationship of the external, objective events to the internal, subjective experience (ie, as informed by prior memory traces, intrapsychic conflicts, and psychological defenses) is often neglected. The discrepancy between external and internal or psychic reality in relation to what was said and done can impair patients' and the medical-surgical team's understanding of each others' reactions. Indeed, when we investigated the medical records and inquired about the cardiac event that Angelica recalled, there were no traces anywhere. One can well wonder if after anesthesia, there might have been a moment of concern that was exaggerated in her mind given a lack of awareness of how terrified she was and how her own internal conflicts might be altering her vision of her son's condition.

At that point, we were able to explain to the team the extent of the devastating fears of annihilation with which Angelica was living. We could discuss her psychological defenses of denial and projective identification based on mistrust, her own deep insecurity paved over with narcissistic armor, her capacity to dissociate and exhibit posttraumatic stress complete with reexperiencing, avoidance, and hyperarousal that interfered with every aspect of her functioning. Her ability to turn passive into active, to invert powerlessness into omnipotence, and to render the most capable surgeons speechless had been easily perceived as intentional manipulation.

This intervention permitted a drastic change in the relationship of the team with the mother: they were immediately ready to empathize with a mother who was desperately trying in her own way to *protect* her son because she had been so scared that he would die than with a mother they were seeing as manipulative, obstructive, omnipotent, and characterological. As her anxieties were better contained, she could also begin to tolerate some separation. She and Paul were able to have sessions individually, alternating with joint sessions. We were able to introduce a second male psychiatrist for Paul. His play became gradually more complex, with greater expression of aggression and representations of a protective third man, such as a knight or a policeman.

At the end of this period, Paul was sufficiently better to go back home. No decision was made yet about the transplant, which was left open as an option depending on the evolution.

A few weeks later, Paul was hospitalized for dehydration following a bout of gastroenteritis. His physical status worsened quickly: he was transferred to Geneva in acute renal failure. We noted that the mother insisted on Paul's transfer to Geneva, which she had previously always resisted.

Phase 2: Building Tolerance of Separation and Anxiety: Helping Paul and His Mother Find Their Own Voices and Their Own Words (4 Months)

Paul was rehospitalized. His mother immediately reported feeling reassured to be back in Geneva and close to the specialists that knew Paul and his disease. She reported feeling thrown off by how quickly, following a happy return home, Paul's health could turn for the worse and how she could suddenly feel so alone and estranged in her own home.

Indeed, it became clear that there was no remaining option other than a liver and kidney transplant. How would we help Angelica address this new challenge and how would we (she and us together) help Paul with it?

We could see that within the therapeutic alliance formed before Paul's discharge, Angelica had moved forward, and her defenses had changed enough to allow her to ask for help. She and the treatment team decided to put Paul on the double-transplant waiting list. She told us that she was very scared about what would happen. We reassured her that we would remain available to her and Paul throughout the process. At that point, our goal was to help prepare Paul and his mother psychologically for the transplant.

Rather than focusing on the medical-surgical risks or on Paul's potential physical suffering as the medical team had anticipated, Angelica prioritized fears of sleeping separately from her son while he would be in the intensive care unit. We learned that Angelica continued to sleep with Paul in the same bed at home until he had fallen asleep. She does not recall a night that she had not spent with Paul in the same room since his birth.

Angelica agreed that in preparation for his transplant she should practice separation and work through her anxiety. She agreed to have therapy sessions at a different time from her son such that each would have to experience separation and being alone for an hour. She was able to talk about the difficulty she had just in going to the room next door for her session, initially only doing it if she could see him through an open door. Although Paul did not verbalize his separation distress, when we came back at the end of the session, he was dramatically scratching his skin until it bled; pruritus is a major symptom of his disease, and the response to medication is highly variable from one patient to another. His mother screamed at him in panic; then crying, she hovered over Paul and restrained his hands so that he would not scratch. Paul gave in. Dr Schwab stood back as this frenzied interaction subsided. Dr Schwab calmly commented, "It must feel very reassuring to feel Mom so close, that you can touch her, and feel that she is willing to do anything she can to keep you safe." Dr Schwab then addressed the other side of the conflict: "I wonder if you weren't scared when your mother left the room. …I know you have the strength in you to cope with being apart from you mother when she is busy." Paul did not answer but slightly moved away from his mother's body and kept on playing with the puzzle he had in front of him. Dr Schwab smiled at him: "Indeed you are grown up enough to do the puzzle alone, you already showed that to us."

Dr Schwab noticed that during sessions when mother left Paul alone, his scratching worsened. She wondered with the mother again in a team-effort if Paul's itching and scratching might be worse because of his separation anxiety even though there was a physiologic basis for the skin condition. This shared observation allowed Dr Schwab and Angelica to discuss further how it could be possible that she had never talked to Paul about his illness even though he had been sick since he was an infant. Dr Schwab observed that Angelica tended to interpret every signal from her son as a form of physical pain or discomfort. If Dr Schwab interrupted Paul's favorite movie to let him know he had a session, Paul frowned and moaned slightly. Angelica interpreted this as a possible stomach pain, when it was quite obviously frustration that he had to turn off the movie. Physical issues had taken on so much importance that they seemed to have *forgotten* that Paul could also *feel* unpleasant emotions like anger, frustration with no danger, or distress somatically. Verbalizing this helped Angelica to depart from her de facto idea that Paul had to be overprotected, thus finding his own words to express anger and aggression toward his mother was unfathomable. And for Paul, it allowed him to express disapproval, anger, or frustration toward the team and then, gradually, toward his mother.

The next step in tolerating separation was to encourage Angelica to leave her son's room to have a coffee at the cafeteria and then to leave the hospital for a few hours to take care of her errands and herself. We defined a transitional object that should help Paul and Angelica cope with the separation. The mother decided to buy a plush cat for Paul: "The cat is my favorite animal, so Paul would know that I am not far away, still thinking of him." Paul did not say anything, but in the next days and weeks Dr Schwab observed that, among the numerous toys in his room, the cat was center stage on his pillow. The cat had become a transitional object connecting Paul to a reassuring caregiving environment that his mother together with us had co-constructed.

This process harkens back to what Margaret Mahler and colleagues[21] described as separation and individuation that is part of normative development during the first 3 years of life. In the case of Paul, a combination of social-emotional developmental delay plus regression in the face of worsening illness caused these early developmental challenges to resurface in their importance during this phase of intervention. Despite Paul's worsening, his mother agreed to sleep in an apartment close to the hospital. Paul reacted strongly to that decision; he begged his mother not to leave him with a clarity of verbal expression that we had not theretofore observed. He then spent 3 terrible nights crying for her, after which he quickly adapted to this new situation. We worked with the medical staff to ensure that our common message was given to reassure Paul during these stressful moments. We let him know that his mother was nearby at the hospital lodging for parents and that we would be available if he needed us around the clock such that he was never left alone. Most importantly, we reminded Paul that his mother would be there in the morning. It is useful to point out here that one can never presume what of the medically ill child's individual experience would be the most traumatogenic. In this case, increased separation from Angelica was much more disturbing to Paul than hearing that he would need a double-organ transplant. It was important for the medical team as well as Angelica to understand that their optimism about the life-saving meaning of the double transplant could cause them to miss the fears and doubts about having yet another frightening procedure that would involve more potential separations, more medications, and requirements.[22]

Although continuing to discuss Paul's reaction to his increased separateness from his mother, Dr Schwab also began to talk to Paul more openly about the big operation he was expecting. He perfectly understood in his own words that his liver and kidney "needed to be replaced because they were not working any more." We talked about the early benefits he could expect: becoming less green and yellow, and, above all, having less itching. He was confident that the operation would go well and expressed more fears of the medical equipment he would require immediately after (tubes, injections, and so forth). He was particularly concerned about whether he would be in pain. The medical team and the parents of patients receiving transplants are so focused on the improved prognosis, they can lose sight of the child's point of view, including the fear of having an operation, postoperative pain, and the need for further procedures.[23,24] Paul's ability to discuss these anxiety-provoking subjects was very new and clearly linked to our approach, which gave great value to his emotional experience, wishes, and fears.

Phase 3: Accepting the Need for Transplant, Loss of the Pretransplant Life, and Owning the Desire for Life Posttransplant (Approximately 1 Month)

Parallel to the ongoing separation process that we described earlier, Paul's physical health worsened to the point that the medical team began to expect him to die, which remained unspoken or speechless until Dr Schwab addressed the team's emotional response to Paul's latest turn for the worse. The fact that Paul was awaiting a double transplant, with the kidney compatibility criteria being much more demanding than for a liver alone, it was very difficult to find a potential donor; and the team had the impression that time was running out. During her individual session with Dr Schwab, Angelica brought up spontaneously that she was afraid that the end was approaching. For the first time perhaps ever, Angelica and a doctor (Dr Schwab) could openly discuss how truly sick Paul was and that maybe he would not survive. Angelica was able to verbalize that a whole decade of her life had been dedicated to her sick son and that she had never discussed her fears and wishes related to what it will be like afterward if Paul dies.

To see Paul so deathly ill was unbearable, for Angelica and the medical team. We began to note that doctors and nurses were spending less time with Paul so as to defensively avoid confronting his deteriorating state. Dr Schwab organized a multidisciplinary meeting to reinforce Paul and his mother's needs for proximity, support, and reassurance. At the same time, key to a psychodynamic approach, Dr Schwab spoke of how the team, in becoming more aware of what it dreaded (feelings of hopelessness, helplessness, anger, and frustration with the potential seeming inutility of all those years of effort, coupled with their own fear of mortality), they could better become available to Paul and his mother and ensure at least his comfort while waiting for what amounted to a miracle: the transplant.

The team succeeded in sustaining better care of Paul such that Paul survived long enough for a suitable donor to be found. Paul received a new liver and kidneys. He never questioned where they came from. This question would be one to hold in mind for later.

Phase 4: Idealization and New Adaptation Posttransplant (4 Months)

Meanwhile, Paul recovered quite well from the operation. As soon as he was back on the ward, he urged his mother to spend the night at the hospital, as if nothing happened during the last few months. Dr Schwab was worried that Angelica would agree. But she did not and firmly stuck to the fact that she also needed rest. When Paul suffered from an acute rejection some weeks later, his mother minimized its importance. Paul's weight loss caused by appetite loss was still very central. When confronted with the need to more actively encourage him to eat, his mother answered, "that's not so important. He won't die from starving, right?" She was, thus, newly able to play with the reality of death as is so essential for regulating one's affect and maintaining psychic equilibrium in the face of stress.[25] This was important in Angelica's ability to show herself and Paul that she was able to contain her own anxiety enough to be able to help Paul with his.

As Paul recovered, his general condition and energy level improved, allowing him to be more present and active. He began to take increasing pleasure in autonomy. He asked to go to the hospital playground for the first time. He became interested in the challenge of taking his medication by himself. It seemed as though he was, for the first time in his life, having real fun. This metamorphosis of Paul reinforced the mother's idea of a miracle or, she would say later, rebirth. We became aware of how new narcissistic defenses of invulnerability were thickened in the context of being a patient with a double transplant with all the vulnerability to infections, neoplasms, rejection, and other complications, including depression and ongoing feeding difficulties.

Phase 5: Preparing to go Back Home and How to Continue the Therapeutic Process Out of the Hospital (3 Months)

It took joint efforts with the medical team to prepare Paul and Angelica for their return home. Dr Schwab's worry became how to transfer the positive transference invested in us and the medical team to a different network of professionals in Paul's hometown, most of them unknown to Paul and mother. So, it was important that the medical discharge was not the termination of our work with the family. The loss of proximity to the Geneva team and her sense of abandonment were such that Angelica began to call us with increasing frequency for help.

Although some members of the team considered this to be evidence of her psychiatric condition, for us, it showed that she had changed psychically such that that she was able to hold us in mind as benevolent sources of security and protection. And in this context, we were able to reassure her that even if she continued her work with the local professionals, we would not abandon her but would remain available to work together with her and with their new therapists. Paul's psychological adaptation progressed in parallel such that even when the discussion turned to his future (eg, schooling) during his consultation visits in Geneva, he asked to leave the consulting room to play outside. In some way, he was saying, "you adults find a solution, I trust you." For the first time, Paul was saying in his own words that he wanted to go have fun and be a kid.

DISCUSSION OF THE CASE OF PAUL AND ANGELICA

We chose to focus on Paul's case in order to illustrate how psychodynamic approaches to consult-liaison work with severely and chronically ill patients from the moment of referral onwards can be advantageous to patients, their families, and to the medical-surgical team's care. Our intervention facilitated Paul's receiving the double-organ transplant he needed to survive. We noted important psychological changes during the process with us that ensued over 1 year: A therapeutic alliance was established and deepened with Angelica and Paul; and Angelica began to speak of her own mind as increasingly distinct from Paul's, showing greater consideration of her thoughts and feelings as informed by her experiences past and present and how her thoughts and feelings informed her actions vis-à-vis Paul and the medical staff, even if only after the fact.

She showed subtle but clearly increased use of key features of mentalization. To be able to help to contain Angelica's annihilation anxiety, it was important to enter into the terrified and terrifying intersubjectivity she generated around her son's illness and mortality in light of her prior trauma. Before change was possible, we had to experience with Angelica and Paul the sense of impasse, a feeling that we were not able to make use of our own mentalizing capacity during the early phase of our work with her (Rusconi

Serpa and colleagues, 2009).[26] Only then did Angelica begin to use less frequently projective-introjective defenses and denial in her interactions with others, gradually replacing these more primitive defenses with a more idealizing-than-devaluing, dependent-compliant stance, with increasing identification with us and the medical staff. The coherence in her narrative of her traumatic life events before and after Paul's birth became more coherent. The sum of these changes noted in the case of Angelica altered Paul's caregiving environment enough to allow him to own his desires and fears, regulate his own affect, and behave in a manner more consistent with his development.

Although this work is by no means psychoanalysis, the elements of transference and countertransference, as well as understanding psychic structure (such as mental representations and defense mechanisms), were in our minds during every interaction and were crucial to the therapeutic process observed. Also consistent with the analytic method is the depth to which the clinician gets to know in detail the patients' and their families' history, with particular emphasis on attachment relationships and prior trauma. Less psychodynamic approaches often focus on the issues that led to referral or on the evaluation and treatment of symptoms.

The case illustrates how our intervention helped the family and the medical team to collaborate more effectively. Indeed, our goal was to allow the family and medical team to identify common goals, shared emotions, and areas of empathic resonance. To reach that goal, we worked on containing reciprocal anxieties, challenging distorted mental representations, and modeling mutually comprehensible language to allow each to understand the wishes and fears of the other. This effort involved using our own thoughts and feelings to integrate the various fragments of experience, momentary reactions, and projections-introjections that would allow for progress in their collaboration. And, thus, although we could imagine ourselves within the system we were observing, we strived also to look from outside the system as an "analytic third".[1]

We cannot emphasize enough that our foremost intervention goal was to build and maintain a therapeutic alliance to facilitate adherence to Paul's *somatic* treatment. Achieving psychic change and a change in their relationship was a secondary goal. It may well be artificial to separate these goals because they were realized in tandem, but what we want to emphasize here is that in contrast to typical outpatient psychotherapy, it was not a complaint or concern by the patient, family, or teachers that was the focus. Nevertheless, it is quite frequent in consult-liaison work that by *experiencing symptomatic relief and improvement in functioning and relationships with important others,* patients and families slowly develop an interest in and a request for ongoing psychotherapy following discharge.

One major challenge in applying the psychodynamic approach to consult-liaison work with severely ill patients is the impossibility of maintaining the therapeutic frame. Indeed, numerous major but also minor events can affect the patients' daily schedule (and the therapist's) in often haphazard ways: medical-surgical interventions, tests, transfers to an intensive care unit, or simply unexpected visitors or changes in course. The next day is usually unforeseeable even though we plan as if it were, and this is also the case for predicting the length of the hospital stay or the patients' ability mentally and physically to maintain engagement in the process. This situation means that we need to keep in mind both our long-term goals but also the everyday challenges, uncertainties, and unexpected events that can affect the therapeutic process at any time.

To achieve this challenging but fascinating work with patients and their families, who are generally not requesting assessment or intervention, we need to rely on a very explicitly presented, respectful, and trusting relationship with the medical-surgical team. This latter relationship was clearly strengthened by our mutual experience in the case of Paul and Angelica, which in turn will benefit our work with subsequent patients.

From the institutional perspective, we find it essential to have the mental health team as integrated as possible with the medical-surgical team so as to form a comprehensive care team. This integration reduces the stigma and likelihood of fragmentation of care and the perpetuation of primitive defenses on either side (ie, splitting, projection-introjection, projective identification, denial) that can increase suffering and dysfunction and even endanger the patients. The urgency of our intervention is such that we cannot afford to wait until the medical team convinces the patient that a consultation might be helpful, and we cannot wait until patients ask for it. As we have learned from infant mental health models (Schechter & Willheim, 2009)[27] and as illustrated by the case of Paul and Angelica, patients in a medical setting are not the only patients. The number of patients in the context of chronic illness is multiplied at least threefold to become the child or adolescent, the parents, and their relationships. As such, from the moment there is a diagnosis or a specific high-risk intervention is needed, the parent-child relationship can help or hinder prospects for positive outcomes.

TOWARD EMPIRICALLY BASED PSYCHODYNAMIC ASSESSMENT AND INTERVENTION IN THE CONSULT-LIAISON SETTING

Little is known about how parental functioning affects the child's understanding of and adaptation to the challenges of illness. We, therefore, designed a clinical research project to understand how parents' narrative coherence and their capacity for mentalization are challenged by the communication of their child's diagnosis and treatment needs, and how measures of parental narrative coherence and mentalization might influence adherence to medical treatment and physical health outcomes.

The goal of this research is to develop clinical interventions within the consult-liaison setting that address parental traumatic stress and strengthen mentalization to increase the emotional availability of the parents to their ill child. In the current study, we wanted to create a standardized assessment of parental capacity for mentalization when focusing on the child's illness and treatment, which includes assessment of the parents' life events and severity of traumatic stress. Indeed, parental posttraumatic stress disorder (PTSD) in reaction to pediatric solid organ transplant need and surgery has been shown to affect nearly 40% of the families in one study related to pediatric heart transplant.[28] We have, thus, begun to apply our protocol to the evaluation and follow-up of patients and their families who return for posttransplant evaluations in an effort to understand what might predict outcomes, in particular parental PTSD, parenting stress, and mentalization.

To this end, we developed a semistructured clinical interview that depends on parental narrative entitled the Announcement of Transplant Questionnaire (QAT). Given to mothers and fathers in separate sessions, this measure assesses how, when, and if a given parent spoke to their child about their disease and its diagnosis and treatment, including the transplant. The narrative from this measure can be coded using the Reflective Functioning Scale,[2,3] and we can compare this measure to the classification of the reaction to the medical diagnosis on the Reaction to Diagnosis Interview[23,24] (Marvin & Pianta, 1996; Pianta & Marvin, 1996) so as to understand how responses might converge with features of the parents' state of resolution with respect to their history of trauma in the context of their own attachment. We can also examine responses in the context of the degree of parental traumatic stress, parenting stress more generally, and perceived social support.

Although detailing methodology and quantitative findings are beyond the scope of this article, we present here a brief vignette of Jacques and Clarice that, in strong contrast to the case of Paul and Angelica, illustrates the value of psychodynamically oriented measurement in the evaluation of chronically ill patients and their caregivers. Moreover, this vignettes illustrates that the assessment of risk should not depend simply on the content of the history; for example, a history of illness or loss in the family does not necessarily become an obstacle to adaptation to the child's illness in the present.

Dr Schwab interviewed Clarice, the 39-year-old mother of Jacques (age 9 years), 8 years after his liver transplant. Clarice was noted as having minimal symptoms of post-traumatic stress. She reported little parenting stress and reported that she had adequate social-emotional support from her husband, friends, and extended family. This state was despite the fact that she had had several traumatic life experiences, including the death of 2 of her own children in infancy and 2 of her surviving 4 children had been diagnosed with chronic illness. She has never been in psychotherapy herself but informed us that she and her family eagerly contacted a child psychiatrist to intervene when it became clear her child would need a liver transplant. She was noted as open and accepting of psychological help for her child.

Her narrative on the QAT revealed an early interest by both parents in preparing Jacques for his transplant at a pace adapted to Jacques' development, without forcing the information. Even if Jacques had been an infant at the time of the transplant, both parents thought that it would be necessary to talk about the transplant soon after the surgery. As Jacques grew and opportunities arose during the course of his daily routine, his parents provided him with more information and welcomed his curiosity. Clarice remembered talking to Jacques about why he had a scar on his tummy during bath-time when he was 3 years old.

Clarice showed a high level of parental reflective functioning, clearly able to differentiate her feelings as a parent from those of her child (very unlike the situation of Paul and his mother). She also demonstrated the ability to look back and wonder about her feelings, thoughts, and behavior with Jacques in an open way. For example, she reported that maybe she had not correctly interpreted Jacques' signals at the time of the transplant as much as she tried.

SUMMARY

We present our clinical work with Paul and his mother Angelica and, in the context of an ongoing research project, the case vignette of Jacques and his mother Clarice to illustrate how psychodynamic thinking during the evaluation and intervention with chronically ill patients with liver transplants and their traumatically stressed parents can be both life saving and permit further emotional growth. Identifying risk and resilience in the face of life-endangering illness is not so much dependent on the fact that the patients and their families have experienced traumatic life events but rather the meaning that is made of them within developmental and relational contexts.

In summary, we have emphasized in the present article the following defining characteristics of the psychodynamic approaches to consult-liaison work with pediatric patients and their families:

- Prioritizing the formation and maintenance of a therapeutic alliance with the child and parents
- Assessment, modeling, and support of parental mentalization (ie, reflective functioning)
- Assessment of the child's capacity to mentalize
- Assessment of the child's and parents' abilities to regulate affect, anxiety, aggression, and attention
- Modeling and support of linking somatic and mental states

- Modeling and support of the medical team's empathic understanding of the child's and parents' perspectives
- Focus on the individual rather than the pathologic condition
- Identifying transference and countertransference elements versus real relationship elements in the therapeutic work
- Observation, following, and clarifying the child's and family's affective communication
- Observation, following, and clarifying the associations of the child and family
- Assessment, modeling, and support of symbolic play (with play materials, words, ideas, role play, drawing)
- Clarification of fears, wishes, conflicts and discrepancies, discontinuities
- Assessment and clarification of psychological defenses
- Co-construction of the life narrative of the child and family during sessions, paying attention to continuity and discontinuity, with specific attention to the child's experience of illness, diagnosis, interventions, and prognosis
- Observation of attachment representations and behaviors in dyadic and triadic configurations
- Active but sensitive confrontation of avoided affects once a therapeutic alliance has been established

ACKNOWLEDGMENTS

The authors would like to thank the following individuals for their support of the work described in this article: Dr Valerie McLin; Professors Dominique Belli, François Ansermet, and Barbara Wildhaber; Dominik Moser and Michael Walker; the staff of the Hôpitaux Universitaires de Genève (HUG) Liver Transplant Team; and, most importantly, the patients and families of the HUG Liver Transplant Team. Daniel Schechter and Sandra Rusconi Serpa's research efforts on parental traumatic stress are in large part supported by the National Centre of Competence in Research, the Synaptic Basis of Psychiatric Disorders (NCCR SYNAPSY), Swiss National Science Foundation.

REFERENCES

1. Ogden TH. Reconsidering three aspects of psychoanalytic technique. Int J Psychoanal 1996;77(Pt 5):883–99.
2. Fonagy P, Steele H, Steele M. Maternal representations of attachment during pregnancy predict the organization of infant-mother attachment at one year of age. Child Dev 1991;62(5):891–905.
3. Slade A, Grienenberger J, Bernbach E, et al. Maternal reflective functioning, attachment, and the transmission gap: a preliminary study. Attach Hum Dev 2005;7(3): 283–98.
4. Fonagy P, Gergely G, Jurist EL, et al. Affect regulation, mentalization and the development of the self. New York: Other Press; 2002.
5. Schechter DS, Coots T, Zeanah C, et al. Maternal mental representations of the child in an inner-city clinical sample: violence-related posttraumatic stress and reflective functioning. Attach Hum Dev 2005;7(3):313–31.
6. Coates S, Schechter D. Preschoolers' traumatic stress post-9/11: relational and developmental perspectives. Psychiatr Clin North Am 2004;27(3):473–89.
7. Leuzinger-Bohleber M. Biographical truths and their clinical consequences: understanding 'embodied memories' in a third psychoanalysis with a traumatized patient recovered from severe poliomyelitis. Int J Psychoanal 2008;89(6):1165–87.

8. Varela F, Thompson E, Rosch E. The embodied mind: cognitive science and human experience. Cambridge (MA): The MIT Press; 1991.
9. Shai D, Belsky J. Parental embodied mentalizing: let's be explicit about what we mean by implicit. Child Dev Perspectives 2011;5(3):187–8.
10. Viederman M. The psychodynamic life narrative: a psychotherapeutic intervention useful in crisis situations. Psychiatry 1983;46(3):236–46.
11. Moran G, Fonagy P, Kurtz A, et al. A controlled study of psychoanalytic treatment of brittle diabetes. J Am Acad Child Adolesc Psychiatry 1991;30(6):926–35.
12. Alderfer MA, Navsaria N, Kazak AE. Family functioning and posttraumatic stress disorder in adolescent survivors of childhood cancer. J Fam Psychol 2009;23(5): 717–25.
13. Davydow DS, Richardson LP, Zatzick DF, et al. Psychiatric morbidity in pediatric critical illness survivors: a comprehensive review of the literature. Arch Pediatr Adolesc Med 2010;164(4):377–85.
14. Schechter DS, Zeanah CH Jr, Myers MM, et al. Psychobiological dysregulation in violence-exposed mothers: salivary cortisol of mothers with very young children pre- and post-separation stress. Bull Menninger Clin 2004;68(4):319–36.
15. Schechter DS, Coates SW, Kaminer T, et al. Distorted maternal mental representations and atypical behavior in a clinical sample of violence-exposed mothers and their toddlers. J Trauma Dissociation 2008;9(2):123–47.
16. Jaunay E, Consoli A, Greenfield B, et al. Treatment refusal in adolescents with severe chronic illness and borderline personality disorder. J Can Acad Child Adolesc Psychiatry 2006;15(3):135–42.
17. Shaw RJ, Palmer L, Blasey C, et al. A typology of non-adherence in pediatric renal transplant recipients. Pediatr Transplant 2003;7(6):489–93.
18. Adam R, Karam V, Delvart V, et al. Evolution of indications and results of liver transplantation in Europe. A report from the European Liver Transplant Registry (ELTR). J Hepatol 2012;57(3):675–88.
19. Bion W. A theory of thinking. Second thoughts. London: Heinemann; 1967.
20. Bion W. Attacks on linking. Int J Psychoanal 1959;40(5–6):308.
21. Mahler MS, Pine F, Bergman A. The psychological birth of the human infant: symbiosis and individuation. New York: Basic Books; 1975.
22. Shemesh E, Annunziato RA, Yehuda R, et al. Childhood abuse, nonadherence, and medical outcome in pediatric liver transplant recipients. J Am Acad Child Adolesc Psychiatry 2007;46(10):1280–9.
23. Marivn R, Pianta RC. Mothers' reaction to their child's diagnosis: relations with security of attachment. J Clin Child Psychol 1996;25(4):436–45.
24. Pianta R, Marvin R. Mothers' resolution of their children's diagnosis: organized patterns of caregiving representations. Infant Ment Health J 1996;17(3):239–56.
25. Fonagy P, Target M. Playing with reality: I. Theory of mind and the normal development of psychic reality. Int J Psychoanal 1996;77(Pt 2):217–33.
26. Rusconi-Serpa S, Sancho-Rossignol A, McDonough S. Video feedback in parent-infant treatments. Child Adolesc Psychiatr Clin N Am 2009;18(3):735–51.
27. Schechter DS, Willheim E. When parenting becomes unthinkable: intervening with traumatized parents and their toddlers. J Am Acad Child Adolesc Psychiatry 2009;48(3):249–53.
28. Farley LM, DeMaso DR, D'Angelo E, et al. Parenting stress and parental post-traumatic stress disorder in families after pediatric heart transplantation. J Heart Lung Transplant 2007;26(2):120–6.

Index

Note: Page numbers of article titles are in **boldface** type.

Child Adolesc Psychiatric Clin N Am 22 (2013) 141–148
http://dx.doi.org/10.1016/S1056-4993(12)00119-8 childpsych.theclinics.com

B

C

P

FSC
www.fsc.org
MIX
Papier | Fördert gute Waldnutzung
FSC® C083411

Kolibri 360 GmbH
Ferdinand-Jühlke-Straße 7
99095 Erfurt, Deutschland
produktsicherheit@kolibri360.de